THE PHILOSOPHY OF CHIROPRACTIC

by

Darald E. Bolin

DORRANCE & COMPANY, Publishers
35 Cricket Terrace, Ardmore, PA 19003

To Dona Lee Bolin, the woman in my life whose devotion, love, and hard work have made my career in chiropractic possible.

CONTENTS

PREFACE

A man of many virtues is Darald Bolin, D.C., one who is outgoing, personable, and portrays enthusiasm and exuberance in all that he does. This is especially true regarding chiropractic to which his life is truly dedicated. He is seriously concerned, yet optimistic, about the future of his profession. He is a happy person, one whom you enjoy the fun of being with, and enjoys life and brightens the spirits of those with whom he is associated. He is an outstanding Doctor of Chiropractic.

I believe his greatest virtues other than the attributes of frankness, honesty, sincerity, dedication, unquestionable integrity, a candid kindness in disagreement and always willing to do his share, is his outstanding ability to appreciate, accept and to be tolerant of the various opinions and ideologic beliefs of his professional brother.

It is a special honor and privilege to be able to express my sincere feelings and belief about Dr. Darald Bolin, my good friend and worthy colleague.

This virtue is exemplified in his book in which he dares to depart from the conventional and accepted ideologic concepts with firm and well-founded conviction and logic. In this regard, should the leadership of the profession (both academic and political) accept his basic doctrine, the factionalism within the profession would be short-lived.

Ralph F. Schmidt, D.C., F.I.C.C.
President, Foundation for Chiropractic Education
   and Research
Past President, American Chiropractic Association

ACKNOWLEDGEMENTS

I should like to thank Delisa Lee Bolin and Sherry Parker for typing the entire manuscript; Annette Hastings for all the freehand drawings; and John E. Bellamy, Ph.D., of Oregon College of Education, for his professional advice.

CHIROPRACTIC PHILOSOPHY

Chiropractic philosophy is a rational study of the processes governing the thought, conduct, and ethics which regulate the science, art, principles, and practice of chiropractic.

"... The noblest pleasure, the joy of understanding."
Leonardo da Vinci

INTRODUCTION

There is a critical need for an up-to-date philosophy, or explanation, for the science and art of chiropractic. In the humble but dramatic history of chiropractic there have been many who have called themselves philosophers of chiropractic. Some were greats, and some were not; however, because of them, and sometimes in spite of them, chiropractic has developed into a proud profession.

Today modern man communicates with a modern language. It has become obvious that the language used in chiropractic's early philosophy has different meanings today than it did when it was written. The evolution of communication is the price of time. Chiropractors who take the old-time philosophy literally cannot, in fact, have a legitimate philosophy. The words on which they are relying betray them and lead them astray.

As a young student of chiropractic, learning its philosophy, I was privileged to have the counsel of Dr. B. J. Palmer whenever I did not understand any of the thirty-three principles of chiropractic philosophy. If the language used from 1895 to 1927 in chiropractic writings was confusing, questionable, or unscientific, I would ask for an "audience" with B. J., and he would explain it in much detail, using a form of communication with which I was familiar. Unfortunately, the chiropractic profession no longer has a B. J. Palmer; still, times move on.

All over the world thousands of chiropractors are adjusting millions of people's spinal subluxations. The record shows that the large majority of these people manifest a sudden and dramatic improvement in their overall health following these adjustments.

In a carefully controlled experiment in checking the blood, the urine, the heart, and the metabolism of thousands of people with subluxations, specific chiropractic adjustments were given. None were given any other method of treatment. The people adjusted showed a dramatic change of the vital signs toward the normal. (See figure 1.)

It is obvious that the human body functions better after spinal subluxations are adjusted. Scientific research is being conducted to discover why. This book is an attempt to explain without the barrier of scientific jargon, why chiropractic is so valuable to the health of the world.

Not all of these ideas are new or mine. These are both old and new ideas reorganized for easy communication and understanding.

I know that not one person will agree with everything in this text; but if it will stimulate the creation of constructive thought within the mind of the reader, it will have been successful.

I sincerely hope that this book will be useful to layman, student, field practitioner and scientist as an "opener" for improving our thinking in the development of our beloved philosophy, science, and art of chiropractic.

"We are all imperfect teachers, but we may be forgiven if we have advanced the matter a little, and have done our best."*

D. E. B.

* Will Durant, Ph.D., *The Story of Philosophy* (New York: Washington Square Press, 1961), p. xv.

Total

All Ages

CONDITIONS	1	2	3	4	5	6	7
PRE	77	999	306	57	11	88	42
IMPROVED	65	119	57	6	2	2	2
SAME	12	872	246	48	9	6	37
WORSE	0	8	3	3	0	0	3

AVERAGE PRE - POST TIME

4.4 WEEKS

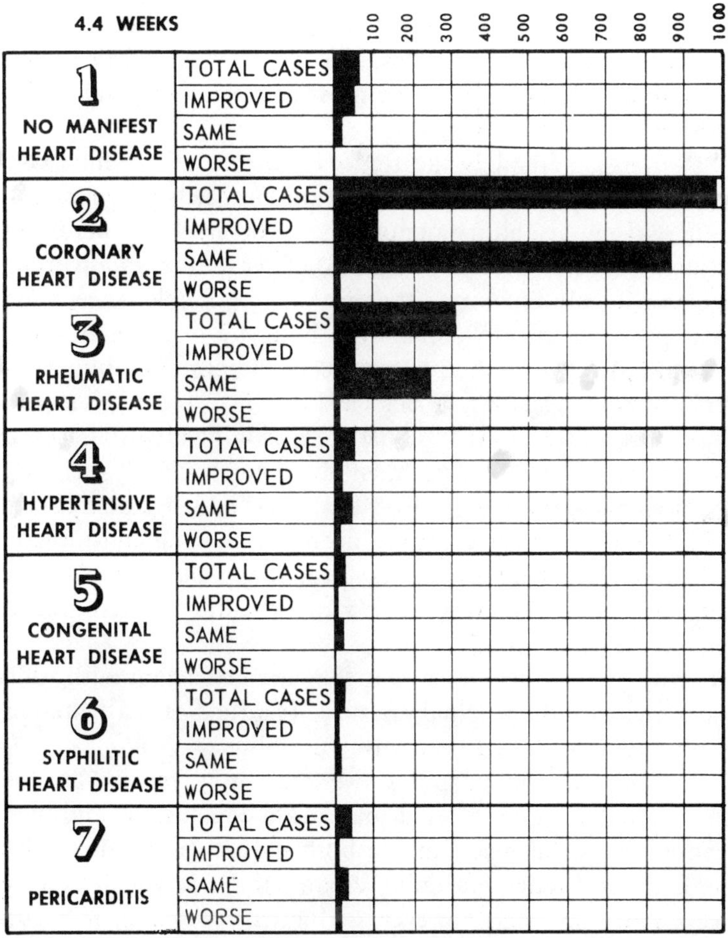

		100 200 300 400 500 600 700 800 900 1000
1 NO MANIFEST HEART DISEASE	TOTAL CASES	
	IMPROVED	
	SAME	
	WORSE	
2 CORONARY HEART DISEASE	TOTAL CASES	
	IMPROVED	
	SAME	
	WORSE	
3 RHEUMATIC HEART DISEASE	TOTAL CASES	
	IMPROVED	
	SAME	
	WORSE	
4 HYPERTENSIVE HEART DISEASE	TOTAL CASES	
	IMPROVED	
	SAME	
	WORSE	
5 CONGENITAL HEART DISEASE	TOTAL CASES	
	IMPROVED	
	SAME	
	WORSE	
6 SYPHILITIC HEART DISEASE	TOTAL CASES	
	IMPROVED	
	SAME	
	WORSE	
7 PERICARDITIS	TOTAL CASES	
	IMPROVED	
	SAME	
	WORSE	

Fig. 1. Electrocardiograph changes under specific chiropractic adjustment (Data from Palmer Chiropractic Research Clinic, Davenport, Iowa, 1949.)

Chapter 1

RULES

In order to write a new language of philosophy, it is important to follow certain rules. The writer must decide which discipline of philosophy is the most complete and makes the most accurate conclusions.

Inductive method is the reasoning process by which one starts from a particular experience and proceeds to generalize: e.g., "After his adjustments, his ulcer healed; therefore, adjustments cure ulcers." This kind of reasoning is dangerous because it only illustrates that which is possible. One must then prove or disprove the hypothesis by experimentation.

The deductive method is a process of reasoning by which one draws conclusions, by logical inference, from given premises. The conclusions of deductive reasoning are valid only if the premise is valid. One must distinguish clearly between "that which follows logically" and "that which is the case": e.g., "Vital functions are more normal following chiropractic adjustments; more normal vital functions make for a longer, healthier life; therefore, chiropractic adjustments give a longer, healthier life."

All premises must show that they are consistent with each other and with the original premise. The field of mathematics is an example of the deductive discipline.

For chiropractic purposes, we must rely mostly on the deductive discipline to avoid inaccurate conclusions and misleading ideas. Science can use both inductive and deductive methods. Inductive reasoning creates theories which can be proven or disproven; however, deductive reasoning, if begun with a truth, will end with a truth. If a philosophy is true to all philosophers, it will provide a sound foundation upon which to build a science and an art.

It will be the general "rule" for this book to rely heavily upon deductive reasoning for more accurate, sound conclusions.

Chapter 2

HISTORY

I know of no way of judging of the future but by the past.
Patrick Henry

In 1895, an incident of world-wide historical human value took place.

Eighteen years previously Harvey Lillard became deaf.

He was in a stooped, cramped position when he heard "something pop" in his neck.

He was deaf for 18 years.

In his neck was a large visible bump.

Fortunately, it could be seen, otherwise it might have gone unnoticed.

D. D. Palmer said: If the PROduction of that bump PROduced deafness, REduction should restore hearing.

He pushed the bump, three days in succession; bump was gone, and hearing WAS restored.

Fortunately that bump WAS REduced; fortunately, hearing WAS restored.[1]

The above is an exact quote from B. J. Palmer, D.C., Ph.C., the only son of D. D. Palmer.

There seems to be no doubt about these facts:

1. Harvey Lillard was deaf.
2. D. D. Palmer pushed on Mr. Lillard's spine.

1. B. J. Palmer, D.C., Ph.C. *It Is As Simple As That* (Davenport, Iowa: The Palmer School of Chiropractic, 1946), p. 3.

3. Harvey Lillard's hearing returned shortly thereafter. What actual physiological changes took place in Mr. Lillard's body may be answered by logic or science, and have since been proven neurologically possible.

When in 1895 D. D. Palmer reasoned that what had caused Mr. Lillard's cervical[2] bump had also caused his deafness, he was obviously using the inductive method. He pushed on the bump until it went down. When the bump was reduced, Mr. Lillard's hearing returned. His rationale was as follows: Force made the bump and hearing was lost; hence, force makes bumps, and bumps cause hearing loss. Force reduces bumps, reducing bumps restores hearing.[3] Hence, we have a discovery of a new healing process.

No doubt D. D. Palmer thought he had discovered a fantastic cure for deafness. The more he examined spines, the more he continued to find abnormal bumps. Some bumps were found on spines of people who were deaf, but most were found on spines of people with other afflictions. When he reduced these bumps, some afflictions, such as heart trouble, stomach trouble, etc., were relieved. The reasoning involved is as follows: To reduce spinal bumps is to relieve heart trouble, stomach trouble, etc.

Inductive reasoning leads one to the conclusions that spinal bumps cause afflictions (disease), and reducing spinal bumps cures the cause of the afflictions (disease). Hence, one has a panacea.

D. D. Palmer was only able to reduce spinal bumps on people for the relief of symptoms or conditions diagnosed by other practitioners, as he had no facilities for, or formal knowledge of, diagnosis.

It then became necessary to develop a philosophy to explain why pushing on spinal bumps gave so much relief to sick

2. Some historians claim it was an upper thoracic lesion.
3. B. J. Palmer, *It Is As Simple As That*, p. 3.

people. Since D. D. Palmer possessed a good knowledge of anatomy, it was believed that spinal bumps were caused by malpositions of vertebrae, called subluxations. It was believed that the subluxated vertebra occluded the neurocanal, or intervertebral foramen, and impinged on the spinal cord or spinal nerves. Since the nervous system controlled all systems, it was believed that any interference in the nerve impulse was the cause of disease.

The reader will notice that up until now inductive reasoning has controlled chiropractic development.

Obviously, chiropractors (so named by the Reverend Samuel H. Weed, in 1896, and meaning "those who heal by hand") were close enough to the truth to survive from that first known adjustment, September 18, 1895, until now. Many millions of people now depend on chiropractic to get them, and keep them, well.

One reason for chiropractic's survival was the effort of B. J. Palmer, D. D. Palmer's son to set up basic premises and developed them deductively. The validity of these basic premises will be discussed in this book. (See chapter 19.)

One question in Chiropractic history that most people have asked is, If Chiropractic is so great, why didn't medicine discover it at some time in their five thousand years of progress? How could medical science have overlooked for five thousand years what a self-educated Magnetic Healer[4] stumbled on in 1895?

I think Marcus Bauch, Ph.D., very effectively and completely explains the reasons in his book, *The Chiropractic Story*. On page 213 he asks why it was not until 1762 that medical science discovered that germs cause some diseases. If there were anything to the germ theory, why did it take 4,700 years to discover it? He goes on to ask why it was not until

---

4. A system of healing discovered in the eighteenth century by Anton Mesmer, in vogue until the twentieth century.

1823 that puerperal fever was discovered to be contagious and why it took medicine 4,800 years to discover that ether was an anesthetic. If there were anything to vaccination, why did it take 4,800 years to discover it? Why did medical science take 4,900 years to discover that mosquitoes transmitted yellow fever? If there were anything to pasteurization, why did it take 4,900 years to find it out?

Medicine learned from a monk how to use antimony as a medicine, from a Jesuit how to cure ague (chills and fever), from a soldier how to treat gout, from a sailor how to treat scurvy, from a postmaster how to open the eustachian tube, from a dairymaid how to prevent smallpox, and from an old market woman how to catch the itch insect.[5]

After reading and digesting the above, it should be no surprise that after 5,000 years of medical research it took a self-educated Magnetic Healer to discover chiropractic.[6]

5. Marcus Bach, *The Chiropractic Story* (Los Angeles: DeVorss & Co., 1968), p. 213.

6. For more details on chiropractic history, read *Three Generations* by David D. Palmer, D.D., Ph.C., Ll.D., President, Palmer College of Chiropractic and grandson of D. D. Palmer.

Chapter 3
DISEASE

Disease originally meant "uneasy, uncomfortable or disturbed." As medical men began to classify these feelings into symptoms of circumscribed significance, called an illness, disease became an entity. In biblical times, the sick possessed demons. In modern times, the sick possess disease.

Since disease is classified by signs and symptoms (syndromes), it has been the main focal point of treatment. No syndrome, no disease. Chemicals are used to stimulate the inhibited and to inhibit the stimulated. Chemicals are used to kill or neutralize germs. Surgery is used to remove an area of disease. There are bacterial diseases, protozoan diseases, worm diseases, fungus diseases, viral diseases, congenital diseases, degeneration diseases, nutritional diseases, allergies, occupational diseases, environmental diseases, mental diseases, iatrogenic[1] and functional diseases. It is said that people possess these diseases. If you have signs and symptoms that fit a syndrome, they are classified as a disease; therefore, you possess a disease, and the disease must be destroyed.

B. J. Palmer liked the term *dis-ease. Dis-ease* was used to mean "disorganized, or without organization," and Palmer believed that the cause had to be removed or prevented (adjusted). However, today *dis-ease* and *disease* are identical, the word is not understood the way Palmer meant it to be used, and it therefore should never be used without explanation.

The accepted formula for disease is $(D = V/R)$,[2] the quality

1. Physician-caused disease. It is estimated that 15 percent to 20 percent of all hospital admissions are iatrogenic.
2. Arthur H. Bryan, Ph.D., and Charles G. Bryan, Ph.D., *Bacteriology, Principles and Practice* (New York: Barnes & Noble, Inc., 1956), p. 326.

and virulence of the disease divided by the resistance of the host. That is to say, if the host has sufficient resistance, there will be no disease; however, to whatever degree the host does not have resistance, he will be diseased.

Chiropractic authorities (colleges) teach the above facts in detail, and most seem to agree that for the purpose of diagnosis and treatment of symptoms, these facts are essential. It is obvious that symptoms, singly or collectively, are dangerous to the life and health of man, e.g., high blood pressure. It follows, of course, that the treatment and control of symptoms is very important to the sick people of this world, and every chiropractor is very much aware of that fact. The philosophy of chiropractic is a reasoning that does not necessarily disagree with other philosophies or sciences concerning disease, but merely points out and emphasizes that fact of the formula of disease $(D = V/R)$ which is the most important, resistance of the host. Chiropractic philosophy will show that anything which interferes with the resistance of the host is, in fact, the major concern, and that the degree of resistance is proportional to the degree of life. Chiropractic philosophy will show that disease is an entity corresponding to the darkness (negative) of a photo darkroom, and that health is an entity of life corresponding to the light (positive) in the darkroom when one turns on the switch.

Chapter 4

MAJOR PREMISE IN LIFE

Chiropractic philosophy is based on the major premise that all life is dependent on an innate, intelligent adaptability.

That is to say, each living organism can sense its environment, evaluate that which is sensed, and react in an intelligent manner sufficient to cause it to survive.

All living things, from human beings down to the simplest one-cell plants must do three things. They must find food for themselves, protect themselves, and reproduce their kind.[1]

Those kinds of plants and animals with the greatest powers of adaptation manage to keep alive when their living conditions (environment) change.[2]

All living things have, to a greater or lesser extent, the ability ... to adapt to the environment.[3]

The ability of plants and animals to adapt to their environment is the characteristic which enables them to remain alive through the exigencies of a changing world.[4]

1. *The World Book Encyclopedia* (Chicago: Field Enterprises Educational Corp., 1957), p. 41.

2. *Ibid.*

3. Claude A. Villee, Ph.D., *Biology,* 2nd ed. (Philadelphia: W. B. Saunders Co., 1954), p. 10.

4. *Ibid.,* p. 12.

Little as we comprehend their mode of work, we certainly owe to the unspecialized brain cells much of the adaptability which has been so necessary to our evolution, and which should do so much for our future history, if we allow ourselves to have one.[5]

Organisms exhibit different responses to physical stimuli ... not only does the part of the organism in contact with the stimulus respond, but the *whole organism behaves as a co-ordinate unit.* This co-ordination is possible because the protoplasm conducts the stimulus as an impulse to all parts of the organism. Thus, the organism adapts itself to its surroundings, and as long as it is able to fit itself into harmonious relations with the ever-changing conditions about it, life continues.[6]

The survival of any species depends on its ability to adapt to its surroundings.[7]

I could continue to quote hundreds of scientific experts to prove the main premise, but I believe the above few are all that is needed at this point.

5. Jacquetta Hawkes, Ph.D., *Man on Earth* (New York: Random House, Inc., 1955), p. 118.

6. Florence C. Kelly, M.S., Ph.D., and K. Eileen Hite, Ph.D., M.D., *Microbiology* (New York: Appleton-Century-Crofts, 1955), p. 18.

7. Albert Szent-Gyorgyi, M.D., Ph.D., *The Crazy Ape* (New York: Grosset & Dunlap, 1970), p. 13.

Chapter 5

SECOND PREMISE

A second premise follows logically from the first: the greater the range of adaptability, the greater the survival value.

Some species have greater adaptability than others. Each species has a hereditary limit of adaptability, depending upon its genes. Sir Ronald Ayliner Fisher proved in his book, *Genetical Theory of Natural Selection*,[1] that the genetics of a species is directly related to its fitness for survival. There are microscopic rods, called chromosomes, in each cell of each living organism with, perhaps, the exception of the viruses. These rods have a certain number of spots on them called genes. The human is said to have some 40,000 genes on 46 chromosomes. Each gene affects its cell by ribonucleic acid (RNA) and deoxyribonucleic acid (DNA). How these chemicals affect its cell is what gives it a Maximum Survival Value (MSV). We can conclude from these facts that the MSV is inherited from the parent cell, or organism. That is to say, the MSV is born into each cell of every organism and gives evidence of cellular intelligence. Possibly, it is this (which gives the MSV) that early chiropractic philosophers called "innate intelligence." The chemicals of each cell, the structure of which is inherited, act and react in an intelligent manner, constantly changing, consistent with the needs of adaptation; hence, we have "inborn or innate intelligence." The MSV, or

1. Sir Ronald Aylinder Fisher, *Genetic Theory of Natural Selection* (New York N.Y.: Dover Publications, 1958).

16

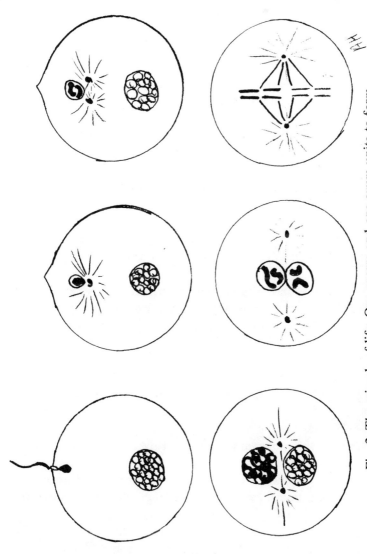

Fig. 2. The miracle of life. One sperm and one ovum unite to form one master cell which contains the knowledge to build and maintain an adult being.

17

innate intelligence resident in each cell of each organism is 100 percent for its species in that organism.

The maximum range of biological organization is directly proportional to the maximum biological adaptability. In other words, the degree to which a species has evolved for efficient organization from one cell to another and all cells to the environment is the same degree of its adaptability to the environment. The degree to which each cell senses its environment and conducts impulses throughout its protoplasm and to other cells of the organism, providing coordinated stimuli acting and reacting in the most efficient way, according to its inherent ability (MSV), is the degree of its adaptation to its environment.

Where the need for biological organization is greater, there is a greater need for cell specialization. The amoeba can move by extending itself slowly, but the paramecium must move more rapidly, and so it is specialized by using little hairlike structures, called cilia, that propel it in any desirable direction.

The more specially developed an organism, the more its adaptability depends on biological organization. The paramecium conducts impulses along filaments to coordinate its cilia. If those filaments are injured, the paramecium can no longer control its movements and soon dies.

Adequate reaction by an organism to its environmental changes is adequate adaptation. The paramecium will sense the heat from the flame of a match and swim to the far side of the beaker where it is safe.

Adaptability depends upon ability of the organism's sensory organs to react to changes in the environment. The amoeba can tell the difference between food material and foreign material. The paramecium can sense danger, and quickly move away from it.

The use of behavior of simple life forms as a simple example is analogous to the use of the hydrogen atom as an example of simple chemistry. Simple as they seem, they are

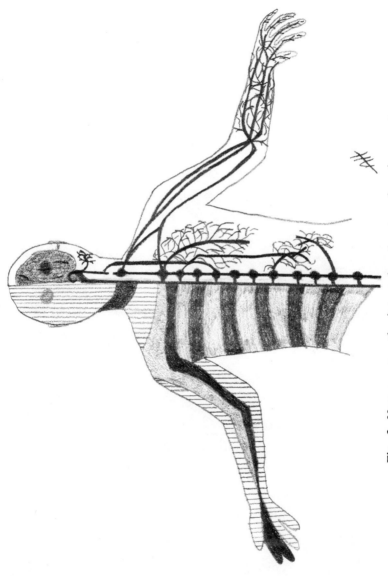

Fig. 3. Nerves sense the internal and external environment.

19

essential to knowing and understanding the immensely complicated study of biochemistry and the life form of homo
sapiens.

Chapter 6
HOMO SAPIENS

Man is the most sophisticated organism known.

Evidently life was created about two billion years ago. The created evolved from a very simple (in comparison) form until two million years ago when the creator organized life into the most complex of all physical bodies known as man (Australopithecus). Today this man knows himself as Homo sapiens.

Père Pierre Teilhard de Chardin, an advanced paleontologist, stated, "Man is not the center of the universe, but something much more wonderful. Man alone constitutes the last-born, the freshest, *the most complicated,* the most subtle of all the successive layers of life. . . ."[1]

Man has classified himself as an animal. Theologians have given him a soul. Scientists usually do not argue with theologians. Chiropractors should not argue with either one. The scientist has classified man in the subkingdom Metozoa because he is a multicellular animal of about 60 trillion cells. He belongs to the phylum Chordata because he has a nerve cord and notochord. Because he has a backbone, he was placed in the subphylum Vertebrata. As a vertebrate, giving birth to his young and nursing them with milk, he is in the class Mammalia. Because he has nails on fingers and toes, and opposed thumbs, he is in the order of Primate. Man, along with apes and monkeys, can see in three dimension at a short distance; hence, the suborder Anthropoidea. Man has put apes and himself in the superfamily Hominoidea because

1. Ruth Moore, B.A., M.A., *Evolution* (New York: Life Nature Library, Time, Inc., 1964), p. 172.

apes are manlike creatures, but he has classified only himself as Homo sapiens, which translates "wise man."

Scientists have placed man at the top of the list, not only because of a creative brain and the power of speech, but because he is the most generalized of all beings. "Because man is generalized, he is very adaptable, and can live almost anywhere in the world."[2]

Man is the most complicated, specialized organism living on this earth. He is so special in his own organization that he is generalized. He is so well adapted to his environment that he can even adapt his environment to his own needs.

Man seems to be a nearly perfect species. If we look closely, however, it is obvious that one of the worst problems facing the wonderful Homo sapiens is health. With all his greatness completely overshadowing all the other creatures of the world, he is the creature with the least health. Or to put it in the negative, he is the most diseased.

2. "Man," *The World Book Encyclopedia* (Chicago: Field Enterprises Educational Corp., 1964), p. 96.

Chapter 7

HEALTH

As philosophers, we must reason that if we are to understand that which causes disease, we must understand that which causes health. "To understand light is to understand darkness."

Health is defined as "a *normal* condition of body and mind, i.e., *with all the parts functioning normally.* [italics mine]"[1] *World Book Encyclopedia* divides health into three categories: social health, mental health, and physical health. We can divide and subdivide for the purpose of analogies and study, but we ultimately discover that each of the three facets of health depends on the others. And once again, all three depend on how they fit in with the environment. The acquisition of food, clothing, hygiene, and housing, essential for survival, depend on all three facets of health.

A person cannot have one without the others. In our present culture, we recognize these problems and attempt to treat them in institutions known as penitentiaries, hospitals, sanitariums, etc. But without the help of his "normal" brothers, the diseased would not survive—only the "fittest" would.

Because we, as chiropractors, are primarily interested in physical health, this writing will not include inspection of mental and social aspects. Suffice it to say that one must be compatible with the people around one for good social health; however, compatibility depends on good mental health. One's

---

1. *Dorland's Medical Dictionary* (Philadelphia: W.B. Saunders Company, 1957), p. 586.

mind must act normally for good mental health, which depends on good physical health, and so forth ad infinitum.

Once again we refer to *World Book Encyclopedia* for this quotation: "All parts of your body must work together properly to give you physical health." That is to say, all tissue must coordinate with all other tissue, one with one, and one with all, and all with one for the benefit of the whole organism. One cell with 60 trillion, and all 60 trillion with each other.

The coordination of the 60 trillion cells is an awesome task, and is extremely complex; but with the use of four major glands, and 10 billion nerve cells,[2] it is done.

When anything (no matter what it might be) accidentally interferes with the coordinating processes of the human body, the organism cannot function to its innate capacities; the range of adaptability is lowered and the resistance of the organism to its environment becomes limited. To whatever degree its resistance is limited, it is diseased. To whatever degree of resistance it possesses, it is healthy; and life continues.[3]

2. James M. Tanner and Gordon Rattray Taylor, *Growth* (New York: Life Science Library, Time-Life Books, 1968), p. 46.

3. The body will not support any muscle it does not use; the body is made up of what we eat, and the food we eat must be protected by us. Health depends on exercise, nutrition, and ecology. To best explore these subjects, read *Sane Living in a Mad World* by Robert Rodale, Signet Y5385.

Chapter 8

LIFE

Life is an aggregate of vital phenomena; a certain peculiar, stimulated condition of *organized* matter; that which is attended by conscious exercise of feelings, impulses, will and reason. That which is manifested in automatic acts requisite for *maintenance* of the individual and the propagation of the species. [italics mine][1]

Life is one hundred percent function; perfect coordination; absolute adaption.[2]

Life is seen in *organized* bodies only, and it is in living bodies only that *organization* is seen. [italics mine][3]

Life is an action *governed* by intelligence. [italics mine][4]

The common denominator in all forms of life is organization. The greater the organization, the greater the survival

1. *Dorland's Medical Dictionary* (Philadelphia: W. B. Saunders Co., 1957), p. 750.
2. Ralph W. Stephenson, D.C., Ph.C. *Chiropractic Textbook* (Davenport, Iowa: The Palmer School of Chiropractic, 1927), p. 206.
3. *World Book Dictionary* (Chicago: Doubleday & Co. Inc., 1964), p. 1127.
4. B. J. Palmer, D.C., Ph.C., *The Science of Chiropractic* (Davenport, Iowa: The Palmer School of Chiropractic, 1920), p. 863.

value; that is the major point to be made here.[5] *Organization* depends on *coordination*. Life depends on organization. Life then depends on coordination. Since health depends on coordination and life depends on coordination, it becomes philosophically sound to say that health and life are the same phenomenon. To be 10 percent diseased is to have 90 percent life. Since organization and coordination are the same phenomenon,[6] which maintains life, we can say that if the organism has 90 percent coordination, then it is 10 percent diseased. Conversely, if the organism loses 10 percent of its coordination, then it is only 90 percent alive.

If you introduce an "interference factor" of 10 percent, the organism is diseased ten percent. If the condition of the disease acts as an additional "interference factor" of 10 percent, the organism is then 20 percent diseased. The percentage of disease could spiral into a condition of death, or maximum disorganization.

It is apparent to the student that something must be done to remove one or more of the interference factors if life or health is to remain.

Since organization is the common denominator of life or health, we can remove the most damaging interference factors where they affect systems of organization. The primary system of organization is obviously the nervous system.

5. It is obvious to this writer that there is no simple definition of *life*; however the temptation to try to find one is overwhelming. It seems to me that *life* could be defined as the *expression* of a very complex mixture of proteins, fats, carbohydrates, water and certain minerals, *organized* by an innate intellectual process for environmental adaptation and propagation.

6. J. I. Rodale, *The Synonym Finder* (Emmaus, Pa.: Rodale Books, Inc., 1961).

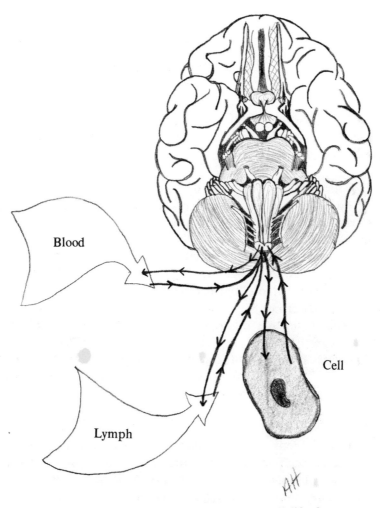

Fig. 4. The brain controls and coordinates all life forces.

Chapter 9

THE NERVOUS SYSTEM

The nervous system coordinates all action and reaction between receptor organs and effector organs and is the cause of organization.

The two chief functions of the nervous system are conduction (of sensory impulses) and integration (of functional impulses).[1] [See figure 5.]

In the multicellular animal, especially for those higher reactions which constitute its behavior as a social unit, it is nervous which "par excellence" integrates it, welds it together from its components, and constitutes it from a mere collection of organs, an animal individual. This integrative action, in virtue of which the nervous system unifies from separate organs, an animal possessing solidarity. *Thus, there is the mechanical combination of the unit cells (60 billion) of the individual into a single mass.* [italics mine][2]

The Nervous System is the mechanism concerned with the correlation and integration of various bodily processes, the *reactions and adjustments of the organism to its environment,* and with conscious life. [italics mine][3]

1. Claude A. Villee, Ph.D., *Biology* (Philadelphia: W. B. Saunders Co., 1954), p. 368.
2. Sir Charles Cherrington, *The Integrative Action of the Nervous System* (New Haven, Conn.: Yale University Press, 1947), p. 2.
3. Henry Gray, *Gray's Anatomy*, 26th ed. (Philadelphia: Lea & Febiger, 1956), p. 5.

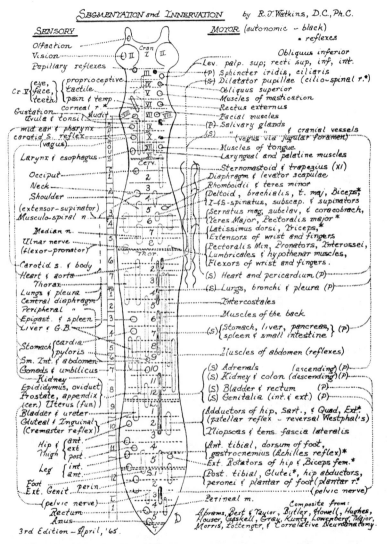

Fig. 5. Segmentation and innervation (by R. J. Watkins, D.C., Ph.C.)

29

Man's nervous system is awesomely complex. Networks of nerve cells, some with fibers several feet long, run throughout the body, *connecting every distant bit of tissue* with the 10 billion nerve cells of the governing brain. Electrical impulses travel along these pathways at speeds ranging from 2 to 200 miles an hour, leaping across narrow gaps between cells, *relaying intelligence to and from the brain.* The heart beats, the lungs draw breath, the metabolism of the body is maintained. The data of the senses are co-ordinated, memories called up, scores of muscles precisely directed, emotions acted on and thoughts conceived. Only a nervous system as elaborate as man's makes possible his more demanding physical and intellectual activities. [italics mine][4]

Dr. Robert O. Becker of Veterans Administration Hospital in Syracuse, New York, after fifteen years of investigation, is convinced that *life* at the cellular level *is regulated by naturally occurring electronic impulses* so weak that they've gone unmeasured until quite recently [italics mine].[5]

Our whole nervous system developed for one sole purpose, to maintain our lives and satisfy our needs.[6]

It is then reasonable that if we accept the premise that the nervous system causes organization, we can draw a conclusion: any interference in the nervous system causes disorganization.

4. John Rowan Wilson, M.D., *The Mind* (New York: Life Science Library, Time-Life Books, 1964), p. 16.
5. Robert Rodale, Chicago *Tribune*, Syndicate Organic Living (Eugene, Ore.: Emerald Empire Magazine), p. 18, Eugene *Register Guard*, April 15, 1973.
6. Albert Szent-Gyorgyi, M.D., Ph.D., *The Crazy Ape* (New York: Grosset & Dunlap, 1970), p. 20.

Chapter 10

INTERFERENCE FACTOR

If an interference factor uses 30 percent of the nervous system, there is a 30 percent loss of maximum organization, which is a 30 percent loss of the maximum survival value, and a 30 percent loss of health (life).

The 30 percent loss of health may or may not cause signs or symptoms (syndromes). If a demand for adaptation is made of the organism, and 70 percent of the MSV is not enough to cause the needed adaptation, there will be a syndrome evident. Hence, we have the premise: One or more syndromes may be present when the adaptational needs are not satisfied. Microorganisms are always present and are not considered pathogenic unless they can produce more toxins than the host can adapt to without causing a syndrome. The host may, however, complete its adaptation (given time, and having enough organization) to the microorganism, eliminating the syndrome, e.g., streptococci bacteria. It should be obvious that the toxins produced by the presence of pathogens are in themselves an interference factor. If the interference factor is pathogenic, the chiropractor must always consider the possibility that the remaining survival values are not sufficient to cause *adequate* adaptations. If this condition is present, the patient should *also* be under the care of a medical physician so that the environmental challenge may be minimized. A prime example of such a condition is streptococcus cardioarthritidis, the germ found in blood and throat secretion cultures in cases of rheumatic fever.

Many times, a syndrome is merely evidence of adaptation, e.g., the rapid heartbeat, perspiration, increased respiration, skin vascular constriction, high blood increases of leukocytes and platelets, and depressed bladder evacuation, as occur when one is enraged.[1] The organism senses a possible future interference factor and adapts in advance. Inflammation around a local infection or foreign body is a symptom, or syndrome, which is merely evidence of adaptation; and though the infection, or foreign body, is in itself a small interference factor, there may not actually be an interference factor of any consequence. Most of the so-called self-limiting conditions fall into the above group.

Syndromes (signs and symptoms) may be present without a loss of health and in fact may be evidence of good health.

All of the above action and reaction is made possible through the integration and coordination of a nervous system which is without too many factors of interference. Nerves "enable us to react and adjust to our environment."[2] Since the nervous system is necessary for coordination, and coordination is necessary for organization, and organization is necessary for life, we can say that the nervous system in man is extremely critical to life. The student must remember that each living thing must sense its environment, evaluate that which it senses, and react in an intelligent manner sufficient to cause it to survive. The human organism uses the nervous system to accomplish this awesome task. Without a nervous system, functioning with a minimum of interference factors, there can be no life.

Let us use sound as an analogy. Sound is caused by an action of force on matter which vibrates molecules. If we are to hear that sound, we must have a conductor. Most sound, as we know it, is conducted by air. Air conducts sound from one person to another, spreading ideas, thoughts, and, in general, intelligence. Air conducts intelligence from one person to another. If there is no air, there is no sound. If we interfere

1. A similar phenomenon is seen in carbon monoxide poisoning.
2. "Nervous System," *The World Book Encyclopedia* (Chicago: Field Enterprises Educational Corp., 1964), p. 124.

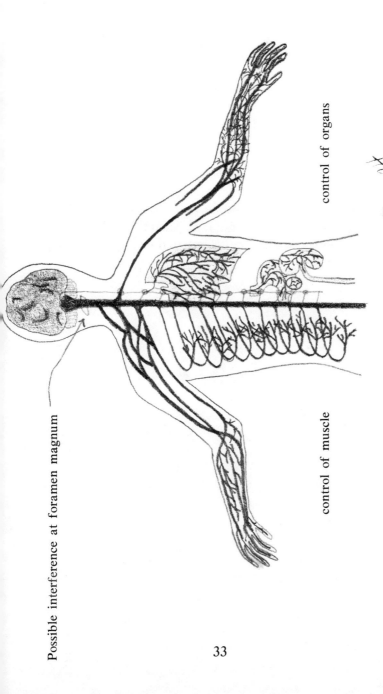

Possible interference at foramen magnum

control of organs

control of muscle

Fig. 6. Educated and innate control of organs and muscles.

33

with the air in the external auditory canal, hearing is abnormal and the message is not understood; the intelligence will not be transmitted. Also, if other sounds are caused by "interfering factors" (e.g., thunder), the intelligent part (speech) of the sound may not be distinguishable. Thus we can say that any interference in the conduction of sound through air causes abnormal hearing. It is by this reasoning that we can say that human life depends on the nervous system to conduct intelligence from each cell to all cells, and from all cells to each cell, causing organization. Any interference factor in the nervous system which prevents the transmission of intelligent impulses causes disorganization.

The student must realize that an interference factor may not in fact stop nerve impulses; it may add impulses like static on the radio. It is the intelligence that is impeded.

Chapter 11

THE SPINAL COLUMN

Any factor that *abnormally* adds or subtracts impulses to or from the nervous system acts as an interference and causes disorganization.

Since the nervous system is so important to the survival of the human organism, we assume that the wisdom of adaptation provides good protection for it. If we examine the human body, it becomes obvious to anyone interested that to protect the most sensitive tissues (nerves), the hardest tissue of the body is used (bone). (See figures 7 and 10.)

The brain and spinal cord are completely encased and protected by the skull and the vertebral column. . . . The skull is supported on the summit of the vertebral column . . . it is divisible into two parts: (1) the cranium, which lodges and *protects the brain,* consists of eight bones, and (2) the skeleton of the face, of fourteen.[1] . . . The vertebral column is a flexuous and flexible column, formed of a series of bones called vertebrae. When the vertebrae are articulated with each other, and the bodies trunk, and the vertebral foramina constitutes a canal *for the protection of the medulla spinalis* (Spinal cord), while between every pair of vertebrae are two apertures, the intervertebral foramina, one on either side, *for the transmission of the spinal nerves* and vessels. [italics mine][2]

1. Henry Gray, *Gray's Anatomy*, 26th ed. (Philadelphia: Lea & Febiger, 1956), p. 167.
2. *Ibid.*, p. 136.

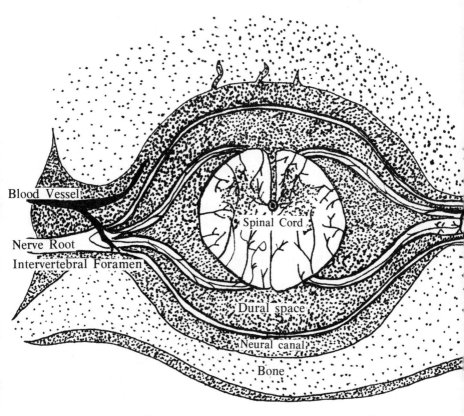

Fig. 7. Spinal cord and nerve roots protected by bone.

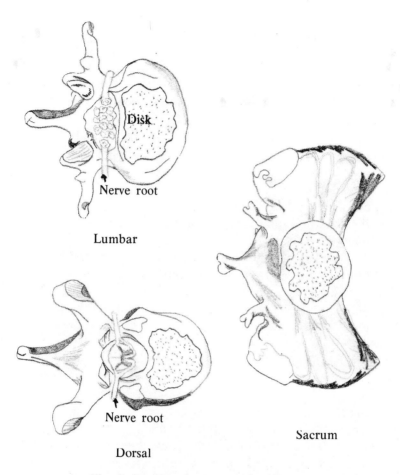

Fig. 8. Looking down on spinal bones.

If there exists a *normal* cranium and vertebral column, the central nervous system is adequately protected.

In man, the vertebral column is erect, distributing body weight in an accumulated fashion with the least on the first vertebra (Atlas), and the most on the twenty-fourth vertebra (fifth lumbar). The twenty-four movable vertebrae are held erect primarily by the muscles of the trunk. The ligaments limit motion but do not hold the spine erect.

For the normal function of the vertebral column, the muscles of the trunk must function normally.

The human spine is an articulated flexible structure composed of superimposed *functional units;* it is clear then that the total function of the spine depends on the integrity of *each component part.*

The *kinetic* spine flexes and extends in a pattern of *lumbo-pelvis rhythm.* Smooth movement of the rhythm demands good *neuromuscular integration,* adequate flexibility of tissues, and competence of the participating joints. [italics mine][3]

For normal function of the muscles (the motor unit of the vertebral column), there must be normal nerve integration.

A *normally* kinetic motor unit *cannot* act as an interference factor. An *abnormally* kinetic motor unit *does* act as an interference factor. "Improper kinetic function can cause irritation or inflammation of tissues within the functional unit."[4]

The dyskinetic spinal motor unit is autogenic (self-caused). It interferes with the neuromuscular control of its own vertebra. Some muscles become hypertonic and others become hypotonic, or any combination thereof, causing the vertebra, or motor unit, to mechanically distort itself in relation to the

3. Rene Cailliet, M.D., *Low Back Pain Syndrome* (Philadelphia: F. A. Davis Co., 1962), p. 31.
4. *Ibid.,* p. 32.

balance and position of the spine as a whole, and the adjacent vertebrae in particular. The inflammation caused by this vertebral dilemma is a vicious cycle and can be stopped only by an outside force, accidental or deliberate. This vertebral, mechanical disrelationship is termed a *vertebral subluxation.*

Posterior subluxations may occur with hyperextension, and result in an anteroposterior narrowing of the mid-portion of the intervertebral foramina in this manner: the postero-inferior margin of the beveled lateral portion of the body of the proximal vertebra approaches the anteromedial portion of the superior facet of the adjacent distal vertebra. *Compression of a nerve root occurs,* therefore, anteriorly and posteriorly near its mid-portion as if *it were being squeezed by a pincher.* A definite decrease in the vertical diameter of the intervertebral foramina occurs, also, with posterior subluxations. [italics mine][5]

A vertebral subluxation can and does impinge on the spinal nerve root.

In considering the mechanics of nerve root irritation one must keep in mind that marked derangements may cause minimal symptoms whereas apparently insignificant derangements may cause severe nerve root irritation or compressions.[6]

A vertebral subluxation can be very slight and still cause severe nerve root irritation. "Nerves may be injured by mechanical, thermal, and chemical means as well as by

5. Ruth Jackson, B.A., M.D., F.A.C.S., *The Cervical Syndrome* (Springfield, Ill.: Charles C Thomas, 1965), p. 35.
6. *Ibid.*, p. 55.

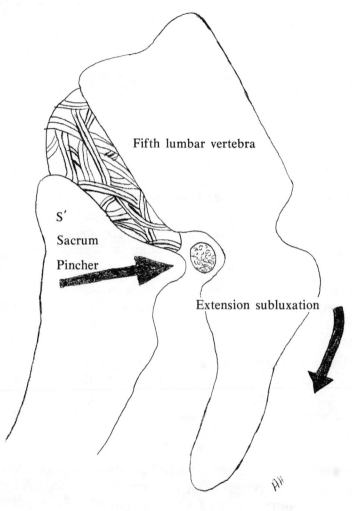

Fig. 9. Neurothliptic dyskinetic spondylosis.

eschemia [7]."[8] The vertebral subluxation causes mechanical nerve root irritation by foraminal occlusion, by hydrostatic disc distortion, and generalized inflammatory occlusion, to mention only a few.

The vertebral subluxation causes thermal nerve irritation by the *constant* heat present (fever) which may be a by-product of the inflammation, but is segmental in nature and can be measured by instruments.

The vertebral subluxation causes chemical nerve irritation by the toxic by-products from blood engorgement, muscle contracture, or the opposite condition, called eschemia, not enough blood and the same toxins, all of which leaves the skin abnormally cold on a segmental level, and can be measured by instruments.

The subluxation causes evidence of its existence by its relative malposition, by its malfunction as a motor unit, by inflammation, by abnormal skin temperature, and by its victim's absence of good health.

The chiropractor must be able to properly analyze the above evidence, using the most sophisticated procedures available.

Getting sick people well begins with every detail each of which must be accurately, efficiently, and competently done. No detail is too small to be done just exactly right.[9]

There are many other conditions that produce very similar evidence. A differential decision must be made as to whom one should consult (kind of doctor), what should be done

7. Obstructed blood flow.
8. Jackson, *The Cervical Syndrome,* p. 55.
9. B. J. Palmer, D.C., Ph.C., *B. J. Palmer Chiropractic Clinic,* Vol. XX (Davenport, Iowa: The Palmer School of Chiropractic, 1938), p. 31.

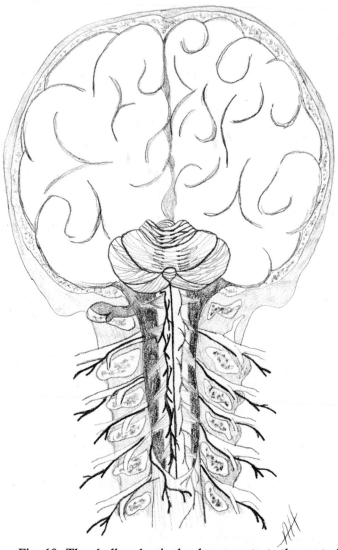

Fig. 10. The skull and spinal column protects the central nervous system.

(method), and how the condition is to be cared for (technique). The following are types of disease conditions.

1. Those caused by mechanical difficulties;
2. Those caused by disease (classified);
3. Those caused by injury;
4. Psychosomatic backache.[10]

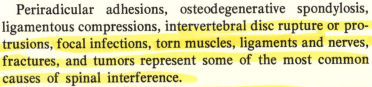

Periradicular adhesions, osteodegenerative spondylosis, ligamentous compressions, intervertebral disc rupture or protrusions, focal infections, torn muscles, ligaments and nerves, fractures, and tumors represent some of the most common causes of spinal interference.

Subluxation may or may not exist in any of the above generalities; and, of course, if the subluxation is present, it needs chiropractic reduction.

The practitioner and the student of chiropractic have come to regard the spinal column and the correction of nerve interference as the exclusive domain of the Chiropractic profession, gained by prior rights and assumption. To continue thinking so is to be without vision and is a dangerous attitude. A rapidly increasing tendency on the part of research and therapy is to seek the cause of disease in the spinal column and to correct that cause by correcting nerve interference. The spinal column is being recognized as the seat of more abnormalities than any other part of the body structure, and is being held accountable for an increasing number of manifestations of disease.[11]

10. Donald O. Pharaoh, D.C., Ph.C., *Chiropractic Orthopedy* (Davenport, Iowa: The Palmer School of Chiropractic, 1956), p. 305.
11. *Ibid.,* p. 309.

If the vertebral column is not normal it will act as a potential, massive interference factor to the nervous system. "There can be no action without an underlying mechanism, and a mechanism can only do what its structure allows it to do."[12]

12. Albert Szent-Gyorgyi, M.D., Ph.D., *The Crazy Ape* (New York: Grosset & Dunlap, 1970), p. 19.

Chapter 12

SUBLUXATION

The chiropractic definition of a vertebral subluxation is as follows:

A subluxation is the condition of a vertebra that has lost its proper juxtaposition with the one above or the one below, or both; to an extent less than a luxation; which impinges nerves and interferes with the transmission of mental impulses.[1]

An abnormal physical relationship between adjacent anatomical structures whose contiguous tissues are eliciting neurological responses that may clinically be manifested as symptoms, signs, functional changes, and morphological alterations of a disease state, but less than the complete disruption of a dislocation or fracture. These subluxations may anatomically exist in the static juxtaposition of related structures or within a point or position of their biokinetic range of motion.[2]

The definition as approved November 3, 1972, at Houston, Texas by the Council on Chiropractic Education College heads and College of Chiropractic Roentgenologists is as follows:

1. R. W. Stephenson, D.C., Ph.C., *Chiropractic Textbook* (Davenport Iowa: The Palmer School of Chiropractic, 1927), p. 2.
2. R. D. Stonebrink, B.S., D.C., F.I.C.C., Dean of Western States College of Chiropractic, *Basic Features of Subluxation* (Portland, Oregon: Western States College of Chiropractic, 1972), p. 2.

A subluxation is the alteration of the normal dynamics, anatomical, or physiological relationships of contiguous structure. Manifestation: In evaluation of this complex phenomenon, we find that it has or may have bio-mechanical, pathophysiological, clinical, radiologic and other manifestations. Significance: Subluxations are of clinical significance as they are affected by or evoke abnormal physiological responses in neuromusculoskel-etal structures and/or other body systems.

The modern definition is only slightly more complete:

A vertebral subluxation is a condition of a vertebra or spinal motor unit that has lost its mechanical and/or functional relationship with the spinal column as a whole and the adjacent vertebra or motor units in particular, and interferes with the normal transmission of mental impulses.

In technical terminology, a subluxation is a neurothiliptic dyskinetic spondylosis.

A vertebral subluxation is found in all chiropractic patients. A patient cannot be a chiropractic patient if he does not have a vertebral subluxation, since it cannot be a pure chiropractic case without the presence of a vertebral subluxation. However, it is interesting to note that in this writer's experience, a sub-luxation is definitely present in one or more areas of the spinal column in every patient who has come to me with his varied complaints, regardless of any other afflictions present.

A subluxation is the major nonpathological interference factor found in an unhealthy host that can be corrected by nonsurgical, nonmedical techniques, and is the most common cause of disorganization in the human body.

It is not intended to convey the impression that all

46

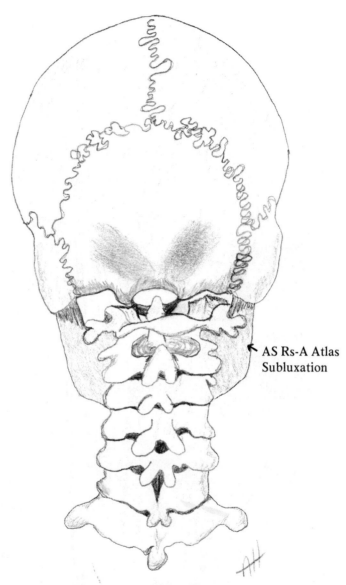

← AS Rs-A Atlas
Subluxation

Fig. 11. Atlas subluxation.

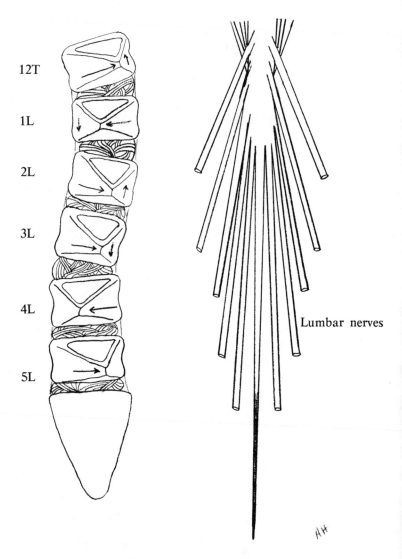

12T
1L
2L
3L
4L
5L

Lumbar nerves

Fig. 12. Different lumbar subluxations.

48

diseases are due to lesions of the spine. But it is a fact which cannot be successfully denied that no other single factor is productive of so many abnormal conditions as are subluxations of vertebrae.[3]

3. Joseph Janse, D.C., R. H. Houser, D.C., and B. F. Wells, D.O., D.C., *Chiropractic Principles and Technic* (Chicago: National College of Chiropractic, 1947), p. 202.

Chapter 13

EVOLUTION

A very important question which presents itself to most chiropractic philosophers is, Why does the innate intelligence of the human (Homo sapiens) allow vertebral subluxation to happen? The obvious answer to that question is that the human spine has not fully adapted to upright posture.

Body weight is transferred from the head to the sixth cervical vertebra and shoulders and to the fifth lumbar and from the fifth lumbar to the feet in three upside-down pyramids. Dr. Lyman Johnston of Canadian Memorial Chiropractic College has successfully demonstrated this fact. The three upside down pyramids must be in balance, one on the other, in all four quadrants, to be without stress. Any spine under abnormal stress has less than normal function or survival value. (See figure 14.)

Fossil evidence shows that the development of the human skull to its present capacity was dependent upon the upright, balanced posture unique to man.

It is my belief that it [skull enlargement] is connected with the further adjustment of the head to erect posture for the globular form of the brain case, with its tendency to equalize length, breadth, and height, is the most appropriate one for keeping the skull balanced on top of the spine.[1]

Upright spinal balance is so important that man would

1. Franz Weidenreich, Ph.D., *Apes, Giants, and Man* (Chicago: University of Chicago Press, 1956), p. 111.

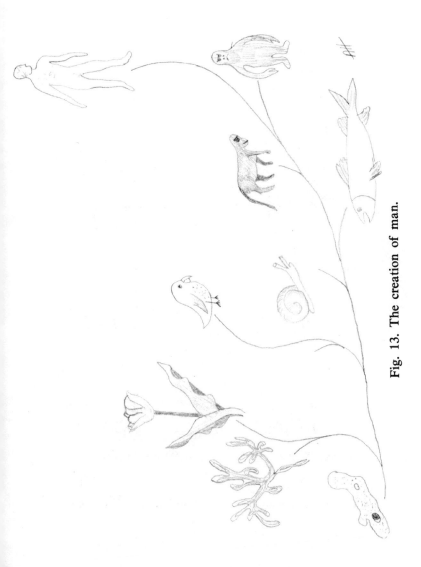

Fig. 13. The creation of man.

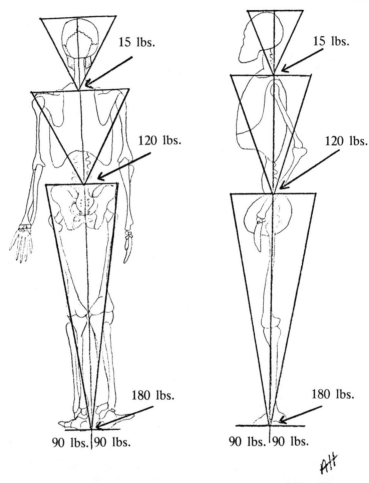

Fig. 14. Three upside-down pyramids of balanced body weight.

never have developed a skull so shaped as to house his present brain. In other words, Homo sapiens would never have evolved had the spine not developed the upright balanced posture. No other animal is balanced in perfect upright posture. Many animals are biped or partially upright, but none is balanced in the perfect upright position. The evolutionary development of the human brain is evidently dependent upon the upright balanced spinal column. (See figure 15.)

If the human spinal column is still evolving, it is reasonable to believe it is not perfect for all its needs. Franz Weidenreich goes on to say, "The increasing brachycephalization is, therefore, an indication that evolution still goes on."

If structural evolution "still goes on" it is reasonable to suspect that the structure, i.e., the spinal column, is unstable.

> The perfection of the back bone and the nervous system centered on it is the *dominant* plot of our (man) story for the hundred million or so years [italics mine].[2]

> The human spine, from an evolutionary point of view, is practically the quadruped spine set on end, a matter which has a distinct bearing on its weakness as an upright supporting column.[3]

Had enough time passed, natural selection would have evolved a spine free of subluxations or disfunction; however, "modern health care tends to keep genes circulating."[4]

2. Jaquetta Hawkes, Ph.D., *Man on Earth* (New York: Random House, Inc., 1955), p. 33.

3. Robert W. Lovett, M.D., *Lateral Curvature of the Spine* (Philadelphia: P. Blakiston Son & Co., 1916), p. 20.

4. Ruth Moore, B.A., M.A., *Evolution* (New York: Life Nature Library, Time-Life Books, 1964), p. 171.

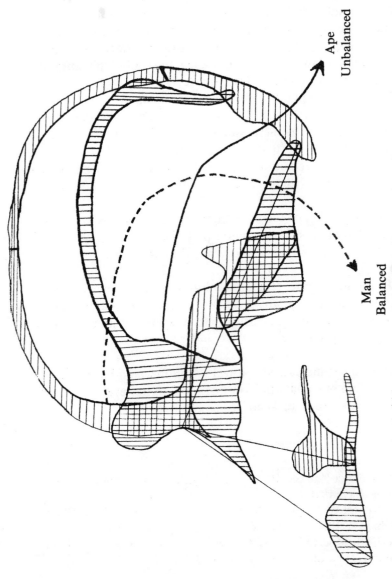

Ape
Unbalanced

Man
Balanced

Fig. 15. The larger skull is balanced on the spine.

54

Chapter 14

THE ROLE OF THE CHIROPRACTOR

D. D. Palmer discovered chiropractic. He did not discover manipulation of the spine or any other healing method. Dr. Andrew T. Still founded osteopathy in 1874 based on the principle that disturbances of the musculoskeletal system may lead to disease and that the treatment of this problem should be manipulation.[1]

D. D. Palmer insisted that chiropractic was different. Chiropractic was different because the manipulation of the chiropractic method was a direct, specific thrust on the processes of the vertebrae for the purpose of removing nerve interference.[2] The specificity of the thrust was the only difference and therefore was the only method to be called chiropractic. Anything else is adjunctive.

D. D. Palmer's only son, B. J. Palmer, was the most-outstanding in the development of chiropractic philosophy, science, and art, a development which caused chiropractic to become a distinct and separate profession. B. J. Palmer defined chiropractic in order to limit it to adjustments of the spine by hand only. Other developers added adjuncts. D. D. Palmer's definition will always remain. Chiropractors may practice whatever the law will allow, but if what they do is

1. *The World Book Encyclopedia* (Chicago: Field Enterprises Educational Corp., 1964), p. 659.
2. B. J. Palmer, D.C., Ph.C., *History Repeats,* Vol. XXVII (Davenport, Iowa: The Palmer School of Chiropractic, 1951).

anything other than what D. D. Palmer said was chiropractic, they are practicing adjunctive chiropractic.[3]

> This is mine. I discovered and developed it. No medical school has ever practiced or used it. In doing so I am not practicing surgery, medicine, or obstetrics. I am opposed to the practice of medicine in all its branches.[4]

Chiropractic is defined by B. J. Palmer as follows:

> Chiropractic is a philosophy, science and art of things natural; a system of adjusting the segments of the spinal column by hand only, for the correction of the cause of dis-ease.[5]

Dr. B. J. Palmer believed that any other definition was either too narrow or too broad. Notice that no mention of treatment is made. A system of adjusting the cause of dis-ease by hand only is chiropractic, supported by all the knowledge and skill that chiropractic philosophy, science, and art can provide. Since B. J. Palmer developed "straight" chiropractic from his father's discovery, he had the obligation to define what it was he developed.

When B. J. Palmer claimed that chiropractic is "things natural," that is not meant to mean *all* things natural. It simply means that all things chiropractic are natural.

When B. J. Palmer claimed that chiropractic was a system of adjusting by hand only, he meant that chiropractic was not to include the use of any adjunctive or mechanical apparatus, such as drugs, heat, cold, electricity, etc. When B. J. Palmer

---

3. A. A. Dye, D.C., Ph.C., *The Evolution of Chiropractic* (Philadelphia: A. A. Dye Publisher, 1939).

4. D. D. Palmer, D.C., Ph.C., *The Chiropractor* (Los Angeles: Press of Beacon Light Printing Co., 1914), April-May, 1906.

5. R. W. Stephenson, D.C., Ph.C., *Chiropractic Textbook* (Davenport, Iowa: The Palmer School of Chiropractic, 1927), article 2.

stated that chiropractic was a system of adjusting the segments of the spinal column, he meant that chiropractic was not to include adjusting other articulations or tissues.

When B. J. Palmer said that chiropractic corrected the cause of *dis-ease* he didn't mean the cause of *disease*. *Dis-ease* is an interference with the conductive tissues of the body (nerves). So the treatment of any classified *disease* cannot be chiropractic.

According to the definition by B. J. Palmer, the adjusting of vertebrae that interfere with the conductive tissues until the vertebrae no longer interfere with conductive tissues is natural, is done by hand only, and is chiropractic. By that definition, chiropractic is distinct and separate; and all other systems, methods, philosophies, arts, sciences, etc., are not and cannot be called chiropractic.

Other chiropractic developers have expanded the role of the chiropractor so that he may use any therapy effective in the treatment, care and maintenance of his patients' health, with the exception of drugs and surgery. This type of chiropractic is quite adjunctive and has lost some of its distinctive separation from medicine becoming a system of so-called natural therapeutics. Most chiropractors today practice some compromise between the above extremes. Only history will determine the ideal.

In other words, any Doctor of Chiropractic who does not limit his practice to fit B. J. Palmer's definition may still be a legal, ethical, qualified practitioner. Many chiropractors have developed sound, scientific techniques (to help the sick) that are not within the definition of chiropractic.

The control of symptoms is often necessary, and therefore, when it is most practical, the D.C. should be well prepared with some method of controlling whatever is necessary for the well-being of his patient.

The chiropractor must know which signs and symptoms may endanger his patient. Since knowing which vertebra or vertebrae are causing the greatest interference factors is vital to removing the interference factors the chiropractor must know "all there is to know" about the spinal column—its anatomy and its function—and about reduction. All are prerequisite for the removal of the interference factor.

Some chiropractors in the past have said that it is not chiropractic to diagnose or treat. B. J. Palmer was one of them. But the writer believes that what he meant to say was that chiropractors do not need to diagnose or treat symptoms but to adjust subluxations. If a chiropractor adjusts bones by a set of symptoms, he is treating symptoms. That is not natural and therefore cannot be chiropractic. Chiropractors must understand what is natural in life and what is not. An interference factor is not normal in life. If an interference factor is a vertebral subluxation or other malfunction of the spinal unit, that condition is not natural. If the chiropractor adjusts the vertebrae in the direction that the innate forces (muscles) are working, providing just the right amount of force, a natural reduction will be made. That is chiropractic. If the adjustment made is not in the proper direction with just the right amount of force, the innate forces (muscles) will resist and natural reduction then becomes impossible. Instead of removing an interference factor, he may have caused one.

It is chiropractic to use all possible means to find and remove any nonpathological, nonsurgical interference factor that develops in the spinal column of a vertebrata (an animal with a spinal column). The reduction of neurothliptic subluxations or malfunctions of the spinal motor units can be the most important contribution to an individual's survival. Therefore, the analyses, conclusions, and methods of reduction must be as accurate and sophisticated as the problem.

Chiropractors do analyze, diagnose, and treat; they must do so or they could not know what to do for the patient or how to do it. *Dorland's Medical Dictionary* defines analysis as the "separation into component parts of a substance." *Taber's Cyclopedic Medical Encyclopedia*[6] defines analysis as the

6. Clarence Wilbur Taber, *Taber's Cyclopedic Medical Dictionary* (Philadelphia: F. A. Davis Co., 1952).

"separation of anything into its constituent parts." *Webster's New Collegiate Dictionary*[7] defines analysis as "the separation of anything into constituent parts or elements; *also an examination of anything* [italics mine]."

Chiropractors analyze the whole patient and the specific area of interference, and then they analyze each part of their analysis. Here, *analysis* is synonymous with *examination*.

Dorland defines diagnosis as "through knowledge, the art of distinguishing one disease from another. To recognize the nature of a condition." Taber defines diagnosis as a method used "to determine the cause and nature of a pathological condition; to recognize a disease." Webster defines diagnosis as "the art or act of recognizing disease from symptoms; *also the decision* reached," and as *"scientific determination; critical scrutiny or its resulting judgment* [italics mine]."

Chiropractors diagnose the moment they make a "judgement" or a "decision," and they must do this following their analysis. Here, diagnosis is synonymous with chiropractic opinion.

Dorland defines treatment as "the management and care of the patient for the purpose of confining disease or disorder." Taber defines treatment as the "medical or surgical care of a patient . . . directed to the cause of a disease." Webster defines treatment as a method used "to handle, manage or deal with an act, manner, or an instance of treating, as a patient."

Chiropractors use the greatest of skill in the natural correction of an abnormal spinal unit, called a subluxation. The "act," "manner," and "management" of the adjustment is "directed to the cause" and is a *treatment* of a subluxation, or abnormal spinal unit. The term *adjustment* is synonymous with *treatment*.

Any other service done for a patient is adjunctive chiropractic and may be necessary for the immediate well-being of the patient; *and if qualified by education, experience and the*

7. *Webster's New Collegiate Dictionary* (Springfield, Mass.: G. & C. Merriam Co., 1953).

legal scope of license, the chiropractor is morally committed to do whatever is possible within those limits, by virtue of his oath.

The "role" of the chiropractor is born out of (1) necessity, (2) availability, and (3) acceptability of the science and art of chiropractic by the people in any area. It is not the given right of the chiropractor to practice chiropractic. It is, however, a privilege granted by the people in any jurisdiction; and practice privileges are outlined, circumscribed, and detailed by law. To whatever extent that may be, the chiropractor is expected to live up to his responsibilities.

Chiropractic *is not* just a philosophy. The practice of chiropractic is an artistic application of scientific principles *based* on a sound defensible philosophy. Chiropractors practice their science and art in harmony with their philosophy. They don't practice a philosophy; they practice chiropractic.

The major *principle* of chiropractic is what D. D. Palmer claimed: a specific use of the spinal processes to correct the cause of nerve interference. How one accomplishes the directive of this principle is the *method, technique* or *practice* of chiropractic and should not be confused with the *principle* of chiropractic.

Chapter 15

CHIROPRACTIC AND NEUROMUSCULOSKELETAL CONDITIONS

Some chiropractors believe chiropractic should be limited to neuromusculoskeletal conditions and some chiropractors believe that the treatment of neuromusculoskeletal condition is not chiropractic at all and therefore should not be treated by chiropractors. This problem is a philosophical one and therefore needs discussion from a philosophical point of view.

First of all, we must define neuromusculoskeletal conditions so that the student will know exactly to what we are referring. The following is the definition provided for the legislative committee of the Oregon Association of Chiropractic Physicians for the state Legislators of Oregon in 1971.

A definition of neuromusculo taken from *Dorland's Medical Dictionary* defines it as pertaining to nerves and muscles. The same text defines skeletal as pertaining to the skeleton.

Webster's unabridged dictionary, second edition, defines neuromuscular as intermediate in nature between nerve tissue and muscle, pertaining to both nerve and muscle. The same text defines skeletal as the hard framework of an animal body for supporting the tissues and protecting the organs, specifically, all the bones collectively, or the boney framework, of a human being or other vertebrate animal.

However, combined terms such as neuromuscular and musculoskeletal are usually used as disease categories under which various disorders are listed.

Neuromusculoskeletal conditions can be considered those disorders arising from the structural and/or functional alterations of the musculoskeletal connective tissues and their attendant neurological complications.

Neuromusculoskeletal afflictions include the following:
1. Strains
2. Sprains—such as intervertebral disc syndromes
3. Subluxations
4. Other direct musculoskeletal injuries
5. Direct attendant conditions to the above
   a. Myofascitis
   b. Fibrositis
   c. Noninfectious arthritis
   d. Tendosynovitis
   e. Bursitis
   f. Other similar connective tissue involvement
"The effects thereof" refers to the direct effects upon the nervous system and previously mentioned conditions and includes the following:
1. Neuralgias
2. Paresthesias
3. Vasomotor disturbances
4. Other consequences of nerve irritation
The neuro-musculoskeletal category does not include the diseases that have as their etiology causes other than musculoskeletal connective tissue disorders and their consequent neurological effects:
1. Infectious and contagious diseases
2. Neoplasmas (malignancies or other tumors)
3. Effects of external poisons
4. Irreversible degenerative visceral diseases
5. External trauma requiring surgical repair.
"Neuromusculoskeletal conditions" are "structural and/or functional alterations ... and their attendant neurological complications." That statement is the "meat," as it were, of

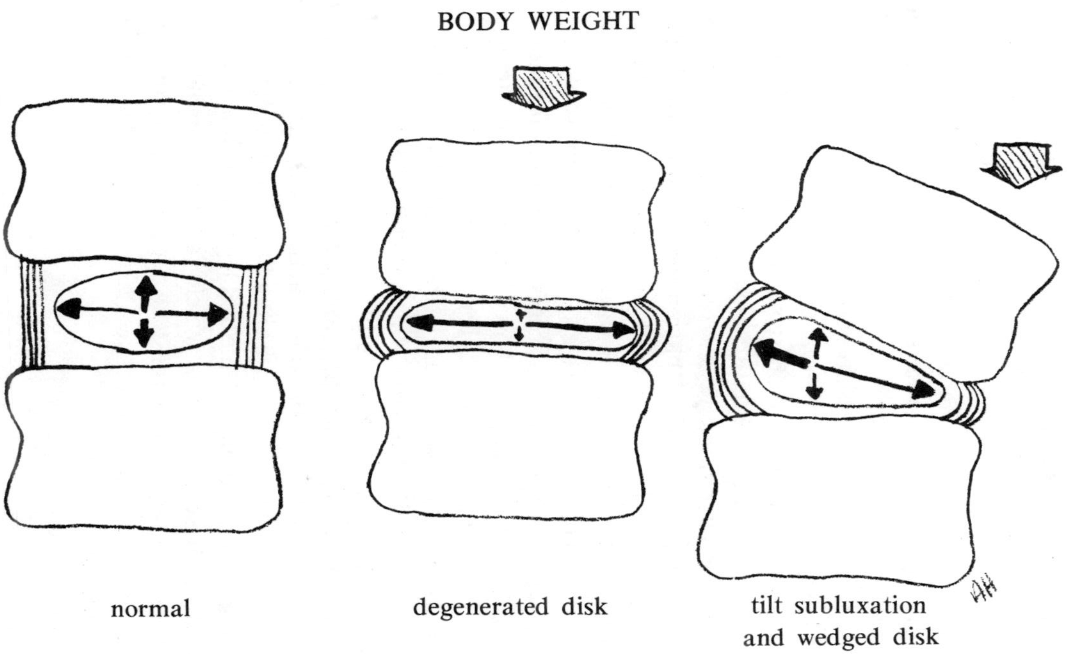

BODY WEIGHT

normal

degenerated disk

tilt subluxation
and wedged disk

Fig. 16. Disk stress.

63

the definition. It could very well be a definition of chiropractic.

The condition of a subluxation is in fact a neuromusculoskeletal condition in itself. Strains or sprains almost always occur in the spinal column at the subluxation. The subluxation may or may not have been present before the trauma; but it is an area of very poor mechanical efficiency, and therefore, the "weak link." Also the intervertebral disc under a subluxation is hydrostatically inefficient and may easily protrude or rupture, causing direct nerve pressure.

It is not pure chiropractic to treat strains, sprains, "itises," "algias," or any other effect or symptom. However, if the subluxation is preventing the natural healing of the numerous conditions in the definition, the treatment of the subluxation is chiropractic. Of all patients I have attended, most of them fit into the category of the neuromusculoskeletal condition. I have never seen any of the patients with the named conditions in this definition who did not have at least one major subluxation interfering with the healing process. The normal reduction of these subluxations was all I ever found necessary to do, along with advice to the patient, for the return of normal health (remission). Any additional effort made by the D.C. would be considered adjunctive chiropractic and might or might not be necessary. The scope of chiropractic practice is limited by statute and not by definition. Philosophically it is chiropractic to reduce any subluxation acting as a nerve interference. To do anything else is adjunctive chiropractic.

For the convenience of lay people and legislators, it is necessary to outline those conditions which fall into the neuromusculoskeletal category and those that do not; but for the D.C., it is only necessary that he, "find the subluxation, reduce it, and leave it alone."[1]

1. A phrase coined by the celebrated Clarence C. Gonstead, D.C., Mt. Horeb, Wisconsin.

One should not forget that the responsibility of the Doctor of Chiropractic is to be sure that

1. a subluxation exists (neurothiliptic dyskinetic spondylosis) or does not exist
2. no other condition exists that may be of *immediate* danger to the well being of the patient (needs medical care)
3. no other condition exists that may require advice or counseling by the D.C. or another professional
4. *all* the patient's health needs are known and provided.

The above is true of *every* chiropractic patient.

The conclusion of the discussion of neuromusculoskeletal conditions is simple. These conditions are either caused by or cause subluxations of vertebrae. Chiropractors are the best qualified to adjust and reduce vertebral subluxations. It is the duty of every chiropractor to adjust as many subluxations in as many people as possible so long as the adjustment is to the subluxation and done exactly according to the natural demands of the spinal unit. It is the need to adjust these people's subluxations and the adjustment itself that is chiropractic.

The student should be fully aware of the facts relative to spinal injury and all its ramifications. Reduction of a spinal subluxation or segmental dyskinesia is statistically the best therapy for nonsurgical spinal injuries whether it is philosophically chiropractic or not, and it is the responsibility of the D.C. to see that his patient gets the best care available for his problem.

Chapter 16

SOLICITING CHIROPRACTIC PATIENTS

There is a philosophical question concerning the chiropractor soliciting or inviting patients on the assumption that all classified diseases from A to Z "respond to conversative chiropractic management."[1] Is it honest and ethical, or is it misleading and possibly even fraudulent?

We have firmly established, philosophically, that all classified diseases are so classified by the presenting signs and symptoms.

We have firmly established philosophically that major interference factors may cause enough disorganization to lose the ability for necessary environmental adaptation.

We have firmly established philosophically that if adaptive needs are not met, an organism will begin to lose its health. The obvious evidence of a loss of health would be signs and symptoms of discomfort, distress and degeneration.

Discomfort, distress and degeneration most always follow a pattern (depending on what tissue is disorganized) and that pattern is classified as a disease by medical science. The sick person believes he possesses a disease and wants the "doctor" to tell him what it is that he has.

The Doctor of Chiropractic does not treat disease; he limits his treatment to the neurothliptic subluxation. The subluxation can and does interfere with organization and thus is a

1. V. B. Chrane, D.C., Ph.C., *Health Within Your Reach* (Montgomery, Alabama: The Chiropractic Layman's League, Inc., 1970), p. 14.

66

major cause of the disorganization which leads to poor health and may ultimately be diagnosed as a disease.

It is a *medical* science that solicits patients to treat their diseases, but the subluxation goes untreated. It is *chiropractic* science that solicits patients to treat their subluxations, with or without disease.

Subluxations cause poor health. Poor health causes disease. Reducing subluxations is good for health. Good health prevents disease.

If the chiropractor solicits a patient with a classified disease because he has a classified disease, e.g., diabetes, he is practicing medicine by inference. What he is doing is only chiropractic if he solicits a patient because that patient may have a subluxation. If a patient seeks chiropractic because he is told that disease is caused by subluxations, the patient has been misled. The subluxation only causes the interference with the organization of the human organism, which may or may not lead to disease. Disorganization is the cause of disease, and there are many physical causes of disorganization.

If the patient seeks chiropractic because he has been told that subluxations are not good for his health and that the reduction of the subluxation is essential for maximum survival, he has not been misled.

To gain chiropractic patients through a promise to treat their classified diseases (unless those diseases are directly caused by the subluxation) is misleading a patient. Just because much of medicine is fraudulent, there is no reason or excuse for chiropractors to be fraudulent.

If a chiropractor is qualified to treat certain diseases and licensed to do so, he may solicit those patients with honesty; but that would be adjunctive chiropractic and not pure chiropractic.

"Conservative chiropractic management" is just another way of saying, "Treat the disease."

Chiropractic is chiropractic. It makes no difference what terminology one uses. To solicit patients with classified diseases and treating those diseases or symptoms *is not* pure chiropractic.

The Chiropractic principle and practice is to adjust, to open occlusion, to release pressure, to restore normal quantity flow between brain and body, that innate intelligence can, does and will rebuild normal rhythmatic energy wave flow to re-establish normal rate of functional and sensibility tissue cell activity to a health level.[2]

2. B. J. Palmer, D.C., Ph.C., *The B. J. Palmer Chiropractic Clinic,* Vol. XX (Davenport, Iowa: The Palmer School of Chiropractic, 1938), p. 24.

Chapter 17

CONCLUSIONS

1. Disease:

We have shown that disease is a classification of a pattern of signs and symptoms.

We established that the accepted formula for disease: the quality and quantity of disease is equal to the strength and amount of the invasion divided by the resistance of the host $(D = V/R)$.

We established that disease is in fact a nonentity as is darkness or cold and is only the lack or absence of a certain degree of health.

2. Resistance:

We pointed out that since we have little control of the quality or quantity of the invading forces of the environment, we can improve health by increasing the resistance of the host.

3. Premise:

Since life is dependent on health and health dependent on resistance we set a major premise and proved it by accepted authority: *All* life is dependent upon an innate, intelligent adaptability.

We then set another premise and proved it also: The greater the range of adaptability, the greater the survival value.

We set a third premise: The maximum range of biological organization is directly proportional to the maximum biological adaptability.

Our fourth premise was then set: Man is the most organized of all known species of life.

4. Health:

We established that health is dependent upon all parts of the body working in harmonious action as a single unit.

5. Life:

We established that life is organized matter which automatically adapts to its needs. The degree of adaptation depends upon the degree of organization. The degree of organization depends upon the degree of coordination of all tissues as a single unit. The degree of coordination depends upon the normal conduction of innate and learned mental impulses (intelligence) from all parts of the brain over the nervous system to all parts of the body and from all parts of the body to the brain.

6. Premise:

Impulses upon the nervous system conduct intelligence, which coordinates all action and reaction between receptor organs and effector organs and is the cause of organization.

Any factor that abnormally adds or subtracts impulses to or from the nervous system, acts as an interference and is the cause of disorganization.

7. Protection:

We showed how the *normal* skull and *normal* spinal column adequately protect the central nervous system.

A normal kinetic motor unit cannot act as an interference factor.

8. Subluxation:

We proved by renowned authority that a vertebral subluxation can and does impinge on the spinal nerve root, and even though the subluxation may be "insignificant" it may cause severe "irritation or compression."

9. Interference Factor:

If the vertebral column is not normal, it will act as a

70

potential massive interference factor to the nervous system.

10. Chiropractic:
   We discussed what chiropractic is and concluded that it is the treatment of subluxations and that anything done not in support of said treatment is not chiropractic; however, so long as it is legal and necessary for the well-being of the patient, adjunctive chiropractic may be used in accordance with the chiropractor's oath and *professional qualifications*.

11. Conduction:
   We concluded that any pressure or irritation of the spinal nerve roots acts as a massive interference of the *conduction* of vital intelligent innate and learned mental impulses.

12. Coordination:
   We reasoned that any massive nerve interference factor subtracts from the total degree of coordination of the body, which function as a single unit.
   Any loss of coordination will cause a loss, to some degree, of organization.

13. Organization:
   It was obvious that any degree of organization lost causes a proportional loss of adaptation to the environment.

14. Resistance:
   It follows that any loss of adaptation is an equal loss of resistance to the hostile forces of the environment.

15. Health:
   We concluded that any loss of resistance is an equal loss of health. *Health* is equal to the *Resistance* of an organism divided by the *Environment,* $(H = R/E)$. (See figure 17.)

16. Symptoms:
   We concluded that signs and symptoms of disease may be

71

evidence of disorganization. We pointed out that signs and symptoms occur in patterns and that those patterns are classified by medical science as disease. We discussed why it is important to know when symptoms can be dangerous to the life of the host and why it is the responsibility of the chiropractor to see that such symptoms are treated as well as to remove the most common interference factors found in the nervous system.

17. Scope:

We concluded that chiropractic is not the treatment of symptoms and therefore is not the treatment of disease. The only way chiropractors can treat symptoms is to practice adjunctive chiropractic. By definition, chiropractic is the practice of analyzing and adjusting a neuromusculoskeletal condition known as subluxation. The scope of chiropractic practice is however, limited only by statute.

Law: The biological law upon which the clinical science of chiropractic is based is the law of homeostasis. That is, that a living thing is born with an ability to be stable (healthy), within itself and within its environment.

Theory: The theory of science which the clinical science of chiropractic is based upon is: There is a system called the nervous system, consisting of the brain, spinal cord, cranial and spinal nerves, the sympathetic system, and certain sensory organs such as the eye and ear. Its function is to control and coordinate all other organs and structures, and to relate the organism to its environment. (Gray's Anatomy, p. 4 of Introduction.)

Hypothesis: The hypothesis of the clinical science of

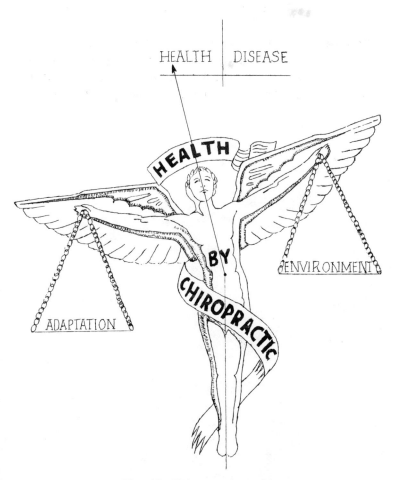

Fig. 17. Chiropractic emblem.

chiropractic is that there is a relationship between the integrity (wholeness, health) of the nervous system, and homeostasis (health).

Premise: The premise of the clinical science of chiropractic is that there can be a relationship between the neuromusculoskeletal structure, and a loss of integrity of the nervous system.[1]

1. Virgil V. Shrang, D.C., Ph.C. Director of Professional Ethics; Professor of Philosophy and Anatomy, Palmer College of Chiropractic, in a speech before the Oregon Chiropractic Association Convention, December, 1972.

Chapter 18

CHIROPRACTIC'S THIRTY-THREE BASIC PRINCIPLES

1. All life is dependent on an innate intelligent adaptability.
2. The greater the range of adaptability, the greater the survival value.
3. The maximum range of biological organization is directly proportional to the maximum biological adaptability.
4. The degree to which each cell senses its environment and conducts impulses throughout its protoplasm and to other cells of the organism providing coordinated stimuli, acting and reacting in a most efficient way, according to its inherent ability, is the degree to which it can adapt to its environment.
5. When the need for biological organization is greater, there is a greater need for cell specialization.
6. The more specially developed an organism is, the more its adaptability depends on biological organization.
7. Adequate reaction by an organism to its environmental changes is adequate adaptation.
8. Adaptability depends upon the organism's sensory organs reacting to changes in the environment.
9. Man is the most sophisticated organism known.
10. All tissue must coordinate with all other tissue one with one and one with all and all with one for the maximum benefit of the whole organism.
11. In man, the 60 trillion body cells are coordinated by four major glands and 10 billion nerve cells.
12. When anything interferes with the coordinating processes of the human body, it cannot function to its innate capacities.

13. Any loss of the innate capacities is an equal loss of environmental adaptability.
14. To whatever degree adaptability is lost is the degree of lost resistance.
15. The degree of resistance is equal to the degree of health.
16. The common denominator in all forms of life is organization.
17. The greater the organization, the greater the survival value.
18. The nervous system coordinates all action and reaction and is the cause of organization.
19. Any interference in the nervous system causes disorganization and lowers the survival value.
20. One or more syndromes may be present when the adaptational needs are not satisfied.
21. A syndrome may not be evidence of disease but may in fact be evidence of good health.
22. Without a nervous system functioning with a minimum of interference factors, there can be no life.
23. Any factor that abnormally adds or subtracts impulses to or from the nervous system acts as an interference factor.
24. If there exists a normal cranium and vertebral column, the central nervous system is adequately protected.
25. An abnormally kinetic motor unit of the spinal column acts as an interference factor in the nervous system.
26. A vertebral subluxation can be very slight and still cause severe nerve root irritation.
27. If the vertebral column is not normal it will act as a potential, massive interference factor to the nervous system.
28. It is chiropractic to use all possible means to find and remove any nonpathological, nonsurgical interference factor that develops in the spinal column.
29. The analysis, decision, and method of reduction must be as accurate and sophisticated as the problem.
30. A spinal subluxation is a neuromusculoskeletal condition.
31. Medical science treats disease; chiropractic science treats subluxations.

32. The reduction of subluxations is essential for maximum survival and therefore good for the health of all persons possessing them.
33. It is not possible to have a healthy body without a healthy spine.

Chapter 19

THE OLD PRINCIPLES OF CHIROPRACTIC

The thirty-three principles of chiropractic that follow were handed down to chiropractors from R. W. Stephenson in 1927, as he listed them in his *Chiropractic Textbook*,[1] on page 31 of the Introduction. They represent the chiropractic "Sermon on the Mount."

The following is a modern discussion of those thirty-three chiropractic principles. It is meant to offer a reasonable explanation and not necessarily a scientific one. Philosophy is a science of reason; however, it does not need to be scientific to be reasonable and factual.

It will be necessary to reread each principle and its rationale over and over again until you begin to understand its true meaning.

1. The Major Premise:

A Universal Intelligence is in all matter and continually gives to it all its properties and actions, thus maintaining it in existence.[2]

This premise is concluded by inductive reasoning based on observation of all known inorganic matter. The hydrogen atom is used as an example: one proton and one electron in harmonious relations form the smallest known atom. The

---

1. R. W. Stephenson, D.C., Ph.C., *Chiropractic Textbook* (Davenport, Iowa: The Palmer School of Chiropractic, 1927), p. 31 of Introduction.
2. *Ibid.*

relationship of the proton to the electron is evidence of intelligent organization, and all other matter is the same in this respect, only different in quantity and combination. Evidence of this type of intelligence or organization is found everywhere. It is called Universal Intelligence.

This is not to be confused with possessing intelligence. Matter does not necessarily possess intelligence, but it is organized by intelligent forces. It is these intelligent forces which hold the atoms and elements in existence.

The writer sees nothing wrong with the above reasonings as long as one does not lose sight of the facts and as long as we stay away from the mystic traps one can fall into by identifying with Universal Intelligence. Some D.C.'s believe that Universal Intelligence is God, who creates all matter. Philosophers of science do not mix religion with their philosophies because it may cause their philosophy to depend on their nonrational beliefs. Philosophies become religions when they depend upon nonrational beliefs. A philosopher's beliefs should depend on his philosophy and upon the facts which prove his premises.

The writer does not argue that these universal forces may be in fact the forces of an "Almighty God." One does not need to argue that point. All one needs to know is that these forces exist and that we can therefore depend on them and use them.

In other words, the Universal Intelligence represents all universal forces and laws known to exist. All matter, regardless of its form, depends on these forces and laws in order to exist at all.

2. The Chiropractic Meaning of Life

The expression of intelligence through matter.[3]

Life to chiropractors is universally organized elements

3. *Ibid.*

innately organized into matter that develops into an adaptive structure intelligently meeting environmental requirements. That fact is, of course, the expression of intelligence through matter.

3. The Union of Intelligence and Matter

Life is necessarily the union of intelligence and matter.[4]

The above statement is again an inductive conclusion and may or may not be true. I see no reason to argue the point either way. Life is never seen without evidence of intelligence, and obviously life never exists without it.

4. The Triune of Life

Life is a triunity having three necessary united factors, namely, Intelligence, Force and Matter.[5]

B. J. Palmer used to say, "Christian Science—always mind —never matter. Medical Science—always matter—never mind. Chiropractice Science uses both and links them together with force."

All phenomena are the result of force in matter. Living phenomena are the result of intelligent force in matter. All living matter lives because of the conduction of intelligent forces. Life does not exist without intelligence, force, and matter. The triune should not be taken for granted, because a loss of health could be caused by a loss of any one or any combination of the triune.

5. The Perfection of the Triune

In order to have one hundred percent life, there must be

4. *Ibid.*
5. *Ibid.*

one hundred percent intelligence, one hundred percent force, one hundred percent matter.[6]

If you lose 10 percent of any one part of the triune, you have 90 percent life. If you lose 10 percent of all three you have 70 percent life.

It is doubtful if the perfection of the triune ever exists in reality, but the concept is important from a philosophical point of view. Any interference factor that lessens the existence or effect of the triune will cause a loss of organization, adaptation and health.

It was thought by Stephenson that only matter could be imperfect.[7] This fact is based on belief and is never proven one way or the other. Therefore, we should not depend on it as a chain of reason. We should, however, look for any imperfection, wherever it may be, of force and/or matter.

6. The Principle of Time

There is no process that does not require time.[8]

The principle of time is mentioned because the student should be aware of the time that is always necessary for intelligence to transmit its forces to and from matter. In other words, all action and reaction, adaptation, or other signs of life call for one event after another. A series of events must occur. The more that must take place or happen, the more time it will take. It will take exactly the right amount of time for what is needed at that moment.

7. The Amount of Intelligence in Matter

The amount of intelligence for any given amount of mat-

6. *Ibid.*
7. *Ibid.,* p. 239.
8. *Ibid.,* p. 31 of Introduction.

ter is 100%, and is always proportional to its requirements.[9]

Any given matter, bio-organic or not, has a certain intelligent arrangement that makes it what it is. If it had any other arrangement, it would be something else. In life, intelligent forces are constantly changing matter from one thing to another until it is used up and excreted as waste. The whole process is caused by intelligence, which is a constant 100 percent for each requirement. Only an interference factor or factors can cause the expression to be less than 100 percent of the need.

8. The Function of Intelligence

The function of intelligence is to create force.[10]

The forces that maintain life are created out of needs which require intelligent reaction. An intelligent analysis of environmental conditions of every area, system, and organ in the body must be made every split second of every day of existence. After the intelligent analysis is made, there follows an intelligent response, creating forces that cause every area, system, and organ to adapt to its constantly changing environment.

I fail to see proof that the *only* function of intelligence is to create force, but it is obvious that creating force is the major function of intelligence. The items that give evidence of intelligence are themselves evident because of the forces created.

9. The Amount of Force Created by Intelligence

The amount of force created by intelligence is always 100%.[11]

9. *Ibid.*
10. *Ibid.*
11. *Ibid.*

82

The explanation for the ninth principle is based on the fact that the force mentioned here is the mental force which is directly the result of the intellectual response to any given requirement. If the intelligence is 100 percent, the force created is also 100 percent; but it may immediately meet an interference factor which would lessen the percentage of expression, e.g., damaged, poisoned, or irritated tissue. A force created by another force or forces may be a chain reaction to a primary action and may or may not be intellectually created, e.g., the force of blood spurting from a lacerated artery.

10. The Function of Force

The function of force is to unite intelligence and matter.[12]

It is force that holds all matter in its state of existence. The action and reaction of these forces is the cause of a continually changing universe. It is force that overcomes lesser forces that changes the structure of matter.

11. The Character of Universal Forces

The forces of Universal Intelligence are manifested by physical laws, are unswerving and unadapted, and have *no solicitude* for the structures in which they work.[13]

We can use universal forces such as the gravity of the earth for our benefit, but we cannot destroy or halt these forces and they would quickly destroy us if we couldn't adapt to them. All living things depend on these forces to sustain life. Gravity, electricity, molecular changes, oxidation, reduction, heat, hydrostatic pressure, atmospheric pressures, and countless other universal forces are used by all life and eventually cause

12. *Ibid.*
13. *Ibid.*

all deaths. As long as an organism can adapt to these universal forces it can live and reproduce by using these forces. When the organism loses its full adaptive ability, it becomes the easy victim of universal forces and degenerates to a state of disease, eventually dying and dissolving into the elements.

12. Interference with the Transmission of Universal Forces

There can be interference with transmission of Universal Forces.[14]

Fortunately, we can alter, transform, confine, store, and otherwise adapt universal forces to our needs. Some are more easily interfered with than others, and some can't be controlled at all, but we can offer some degree of resistance to all of them long enough to live with them. We can best interfere with universal forces at the point of their transmission, e.g., water, electricity, light, heat, gravity, magnetism, etc.

13. The Function of Matter

The function of matter is to express force.[14]

It takes atomic and molecular force to maintain matter in existence even if it has no life. Therefore all matter is the expression of force. Matter is the tool through which force can be expressed. One would not be known without the other.

14. Universal Life

Force is manifested by motion in matter; all matter has motion; therefore there is universal life in all matter.[15]

Life, here, is thought of as motion. The motion of molecules

14. *Ibid.*
15. *Ibid.*

is caused by a force known as heat. Theoretically, matter could exist without heat (absolute zero), and therefore have no life. But atoms always have motion (of electrons) even without heat. With that point of observation, one could say that all matter has life.

The hypothesis created here is that all matter has life, and the more complicated or sophisticated the matter (organic), the more sophisticated is the life. Eventually the matter will have an innate intelligence of its own and will be able to adapt to changes by changing its own chemistry and structure to maintain its own existence.

15. No Motion without the Effort of Force

Matter can have no motion without the application of force by intelligence.[15]

There can be no motion of any kind of matter without some form of force. Since it has been deduced that force is the communication of intelligence with matter, then it is reasonable to say that the motion of matter is caused by intelligence through force. Refer to the eighth principle. However, I think we should consider the possibility that intelligence is created by a force or a combination of forces.

It is also possible that matter creates force and force creates intelligence. Or it may be an alternating process, a continuous cycle, or some combination. The point is that we never see one without the other two.

17. Cause and Effect

Every effect has a cause and every cause has effects.[16]

16. *Ibid.*

There is no need for discussion since everyone is aware of the physical law of "cause and effect."

18. Evidence of Life

The signs of life are evidence of the intelligence of life.[17]

They (signs) are motions of the adaptive kind which show the presence and government of a localized intelligence. They differ from the motions of universal forces, in that they show selection and the judgement of local intelligence in every phase. They meet, use, or oppose every environmental circumstance, if it is within the range of their limitations. There are five principal signs of life. Their names in order of importance are: assimilation, excretion, adaptability, growth, and reproduction. An organism may have these signs so latent that it is difficult to tell whether the organism is alive or not. Yet this low organism has its share, its quota, the requisite amount of intelligence for its state of organization.[18]

The writer thinks Stephenson's explanation is valid and proper. He makes the point very clear.

19. Organic Matter

The material of the body of a living thing is organized matter.[19]

All organic matter is constructed by a living body. It is a living body that gives organic matter organization. It is never

17. *Ibid.*
18. *Ibid.,* p. 256.
19. *Ibid.,* p. 31 of Introduction.

found in nature created by accident. It may be found in the future to be "accidentally" created in the most simple forms; however, we can still argue that it is no "accident." The point to be made here is simply that organized matter requires a living or intelligent force for its creation. We can take C_{12} H_{22}, and O_{11} (the formula for sugar) and mix it a million different ways; but we never get sugar. Sugar can only be made by a living thing.

The intelligence present in life knows just how to mix it, catalyze it, and bind it into a molecule. This is true of most organic matter, from the simplest molecule to the most complicated; however, "Nowadays many 'organic' compounds can be built up in the laboratory *with the aid of living creatures.*"[20]

20. Innate Intelligence

A living thing has an inborn intelligence within the body, called Innate Intelligence.[21]

Innate means "born within." All living things organize themselves into special types of organisms with intellectual precision, following certain instinctive patterns (RNA and DNA), and maintaining their bodies in existence by environmental adaptation. The signs of life are the signs of an inborn intelligence.

21. The Mission of Innate Intelligence

The mission of Innate Intelligence is to maintain the

20. Michael W. Ovenden, Ph.D., *Life in the Universe* (Garden City, New York: Anchor Books, Doubleday & Co., Inc., 1962), p. 111.
21. Stephenson, *Chiropractic Textbook*, p. 31 of Introduction.

material of the body of a "living thing" in active organization.[22]

In other words, the mission of innate intelligence is to maintain life in as many body cells as possible and to keep as many of these live cells as possible organized into one whole living body. One act depends on the other and is automatically done by the built-in, ever-present innate intelligence.

22. The Amount of Innate Intelligence

There is 100% of Innate Intelligence in every living thing, the requisite amount, proportioned to its organization.[23]

The amount of innate intelligence needed in a living thing is relative only to the demands of the species and is always 100 percent for that particular species. The 100 percent expression of that intelligence depends on 100 percent matter and 100 percent force. The writer doubts if this is ever found in nature, because the forces of the universe are always inhibiting the innate forces and bio-organic matter of living things.

23. The Function of Innate Intelligence

The function of Innate Intelligence is to adapt universal forces and matter for use in the body, so that all parts of the body will have co-ordinated action for mutual benefit.[24]

Inorganic elements with no adaptive character are assembled and organized into matter with adaptive character,

22. *Ibid.*
23. *Ibid.*
24. *Ibid.*

which is the creation of life. Life is created from the reproductive "seeds" of parent organisms and the maintenance thereof of innate intelligence.

24. The Limits of Adaptation

Innate Intelligence adapts forces and matter for the body as long as it can do so without breaking a universal law; or Innate Intelligence is limited by the limitations of matter.[25]

The function of innate intelligence is dependent upon the universal physical laws and can never be supernatural, and therefore it is limited to the degree to which the matter in which it is expressed is limited.

25. The Character of Innate Forces

The forces of Innate Intelligence never injure or destroy the structures in which they work.[26]

The destruction of living tissue is always done in the absence of innate control. Cancer research tends to prove the above thesis. If destruction of tissue is found only in the absence of innate control, then the presence of innate forces cannot be held responsible. Microtrauma somehow interferes with the innate control (hydrocarbons, radiation, poisons, pressure, etc.) and ultimately causes its destruction.

26. Comparison of Universal and Innate Forces

In order to carry on the universal cycle of life, universal

25. *Ibid.*
26. *Ibid.*

forces are destructive, and innate forces constructive as regards structural matter.[27]

The forces of the universe are constantly causing more complex chemistry to be reduced or oxidized to simple chemistry (H, CH_4, etc.), and the innate forces are constantly uniting simple chemistry into highly complex and sophisticated molecules and compounds capable of giving, maintaining, and duplicating living matter.

Non-living things seem always to tend to change from the more highly arranged state to the less highly arranged while a living thing has within its own make-up this ability to keep its structure while the material of which it is made changes.[28]

27. The Normality of Innate Intelligence

Innate Intelligence is always normal and its function is always normal.[29]

Refer to the twenty-second principle; the discussion is the same for both. Any imperfection is found only in structure and cannot be found in the intelligence, because the intelligence is perfect for the organism it created.

28. The Conductors of Innate Forces

The forces of Innate Intelligence operate through or over the nervous system in animal bodies.[30]

27. *Ibid.*
28. Ovenden, *Life in the Universe,* p. 82-83.
29. Stephenson, *Chiropractic Textbook*, p. 31 of Introduction.
30. *Ibid.*

The nervous system is apparently the most efficient conductor of the intelligent coordinating messages which are so essential for adaptation. All tissues conduct innate forces, especially the cell nuclei; however, nerve tissue is best adapted for the purpose of conductivity.

29. Interference with Transmission of Innate Forces

There can be interference with the transmission of Innate forces.[31]

Anything that can physically effect the conductivity of body tissues interferes with the transmission of innate forces. The most interference can be made in the nerve system, e.g., pressure, poison, heat, cold, degeneration, etc.

30. The Cause of Dis-ease

Interference with the transmission of Innate causes incoordination of dis-ease.[32]

The word *dis-ease* is not to be confused with the word *disease*. They do not mean the same now nor did they mean the same when *dis-ease* was used by B. J. Palmer. Disease is a classification of signs and symptoms. Dis-ease is a loss of "life" to some degree short of death due to an interference in the conductivity of innate forces. Dis-ease by definition cannot exist without a loss of innate coordination. Disease can exist without dis-ease and vice-versa. Disease is a classification of a sickness; dis-ease is incoordination in the sick body. The cause of incoordination is some kind of interference with the

31. *Ibid.*
32. *Ibid.*

transmission of innate forces. Interference with innate forces is the cause of dis-ease.

31. Subluxations

Interference with transmission in the body is always directly or indirectly due to subluxations in the spinal column.[33]

From a clinical point of view, the clinician can always find evidence of incoordination, to some degree, in all people who are sick. He can also always find vertebral subluxations (as defined by chiropractors) in conjunction with the incoordination. The clinician can reduce the subluxations. Following reduction, there is always better coordination, and the patient is always less sick. It is obvious that the subluxation is always directly or indirectly involved in all cases of dis-ease. This fact, however, is not to be taken as meaning that the subluxation is the *only* cause of interference with innate transmission. There are literally thousands of things that *can* interfere with innate transmission. *Anything that irritates* the body tissues, stimulating or inhibiting them, uses up millions of conducting tissue cells and therefore acts as a major interference factor.

The subluxation is a major interference factor, by definition, and uses up millions of conducting tissues by its existence. At least one subluxation is always found in every sick person and more often two or three are evident in several compensatory areas.

The reduction of these subluxations becomes the most important need for the long-range adaptation or survival value of the afflicted spinal animal, whenever they are found.

A subluxation is the result of unbalanced resistive forces in response to an invading penetrative force.[34]

33. *Ibid.*
34. *Ibid.*, Article 387, p. 322.

92

The "invading penetrative force" is in itself a major interference factor, and if it interferes greatly enough, overcoming the innate forces of resistance, a subluxation may occur which then becomes perpetual or autogenic and produces a critical interference factor, causing a state of dis-ease.

32. The Principle of Coordination

Co-ordination is the principle of harmonious action of all the parts of an organism, in fulfilling their offices and purposes.[35]

Each part of the body needs to know exactly what it must do to meet its quota in supporting the organism as a whole. Knowing what to do and doing it depends entirely upon the "principle of harmonious action." All tissue of the human organism acts in accordance with the principle of harmonious action.

If the tissues of conductivity do not or cannot meet their quota in conducting vital impulses, the organism will not be in harmony and therefore will be dis-eased. The more an organism is dis-eased, the less it can adapt to its environment. The less an organism can adapt, the less life it possesses. The less life it possesses, the more sick the organism. Soon there is no life at all.

Therefore, life is dependent upon the principle of coordination.

33. The Law of Demand and Supply

The Law of Demand and Supply is existent in the body in its ideal state; where in the "clearing house" is the brain, Innate the virtuous "banker," brain cells "clerks," and nerve cells "messengers."[36]

35. *Ibid.*, p. 31 of Introduction.
36. *Ibid.*

The environment constantly makes variable "demands" on the organism. The organism must make instant and accurate changes to "supply" just the right amount of adaptation for every demand. If the "supply" can not meet the "demand," the organism will fail to adapt and will become sick and die.

Interference factors cause obstructions in conduction of innate forces, preventing normal adaptation, so that the "demand" is greater than the "supply." Removing the obstruction allows normal adaptation, so that the "supply" is equal to the "demand." When the supply is equal to the demand, the organism lives.

Life is equal to the resistance of the organism divided by the virulence of the invasion or $L = D/S$. Life is equal to the *environmental* demand divided by the *innate* supply.

No greater thing can be done for the well-being of a man than to remove from him the obstructions to life.

Chapter 20

THE ETERNAL LIFE FORCE WITHIN

Only by understanding the wisdom of the body shall we attain that mastery of disease and pain which will enable us to relieve the burden of mankind.[1]

Life for man begins by the marriage of two "half-cells" provided by the parents. Who the original parents were is not important to chiropractic philosophy. What those two half cells possess and how they provide and perpetuate human life is indeed important to chiropractic philosophers.

Two half-cells unite to form one cell. That one cell is the master cell. It contains all the inherent needs of the full-grown and fully alive adult of 60 trillion cells.

One master cell starts the miracle of life by splitting into two identical cells and then repeating that process over and over again, always giving to the daughter cells all the inherent qualities of the one master cell. Finally these dividing cells take special shape and structure to prepare for special duties in the scheme of life. Some cells become bone; others, muscles, heart cells, liver cells, pituitary cells, brain cells, and on and on until they make a total of 60 trillion. Those 60 trillion cells make up the most complicated, sophisticated, bioelectrical-chemical-mechanical organization of any structure on earth.

In observing nature, scientists are confronted with the

1. Walter B. Cannon, M.D., Sc.D., *The Wisdom of the Body* (New York: W. W. Norton & Co., Inc., 1967), p. 15.

simple and the complex. And nothing appears to be more complex than life itself.[2]

What are the forces that cause such an impossible miracle to happen and with such perfection? What makes the master cell divide? What makes the daughter cells specialize? How do these tiny blobs of protoplasm learn to differentiate, to form special shapes and perform special and different duties? What causes the cells to unite into vital body organs? What governs the growth of the child into the adult, and what decides to stop growth?

What is it that tells the vital organs what to do even before they are fully developed and with such precision as to cause the body to live in a hostile environment for an average of 70 years?

These general questions and many more are being studied by scientists the world over. Philosophers may ponder these questions if for no other reason than to recognize the awesome complexity of even the most simple form of life and "to find the way" of the life giving forces obvious in every living thing.

Chiropractic philosophers have given the name of innate intelligence to the inborn life forces of all living things. All natural forces outside of the living, chiropractors have called universal forces. For the purpose of recognizing the importance of these universal and innate forces, we need to study their effects on life and how they fit into the scheme of things.

The universal forces are constantly at work decaying the universe. This action is called "entropy." All matter of the earth is unstable and is always decaying until it reaches its *most simple* level of stability. In other words, complex matter is constantly changing into a simple form. Never is there an increase in order without the presence of life.

All molecules result from an electrochemical tendency to

2. *Science Year*, 1965 (Chicago: Field Enterprises Educational Corp., 1965), p. 18.

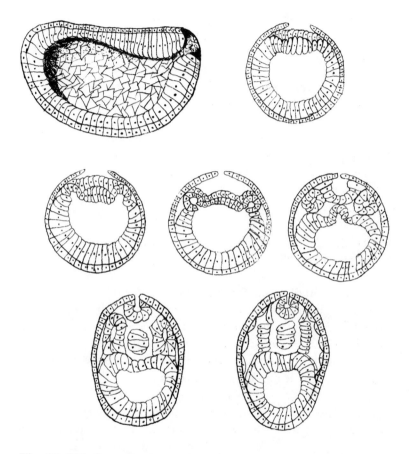

Fig. 18. Life forces begin to shape and organize a human being.

neutralization. Thus it is inconceivable that an organic compound should ever be formed in the absence of life.[3]

Nonliving matter simply does not and cannot maintain or improve itself. Universal forces are constantly eroding *all* matter *all the time*. The more time, the more erosion takes place. One single living cell of protoplasm can withstand the universal forces better for its existence than can the great architecture of gigantic cities.

In terms of molecular structure, a bacterium is far more complex than any inanimate system known to man. There is not a laboratory in the world which can compete with the biochemical activity of the smallest living organism.[4]

To grasp in detail the physicochemical organization of the *simplest* cell is far beyond our capacity [italics mine].[5]

A city cannot stand alone. It is in a constant state of decay and must be maintained by its creators or it will perish under the forces of the universe. That is the effect of universal forces. However, in life, even the simple amoeba can survive long enough to reproduce itself many times over without outside help; and it has been on earth millions of years because innate forces have been constantly organizing simple compounds into the more complex, building up matter. All living matter is supported by the ingestion of other matter. It then

3. *Discovery* (New Haven, Connecticut: Peabody Museum of Natural History, Yale University), May 1962, p. 44.
4. Sir James Gray, *Science Today,* 1961, Granada TV Network of Great Britain, p. 21.
5. Loren Eiseley, *The Immense Journey* (New York: Random House, 1957), p. 206.

intelligently forms more complex compounds necessary to create and support more life, ad infinitum.

The largest single manufacturing process in the world takes place in one of the smallest units of life—cells of green plants. The manufacturing process is photosynthesis. Each year this process accounts for the transformation of 100 billion tons of the inorganic element carbon into organic forms that support life. By contrast, all the big blast furnaces of the world make only a half billion tons of steel in the same time.[6]

The difference between nonliving matter and a living cell is fantastically enormous. The best scientists in the world working in the finest laboratories cannot create one living cell from inanimate matter. Life can only come from life. Even if some day man does find some way to organize elements into life it would only prove the necessity of an intelligent directing force.

Life is no accident. Can anyone believe that one could put all the necessary parts for a fine Swiss watch into a box and then shake the box until all the parts accidentally assembled and formed the perfect watch? It could never happen. The parts would soon decay to dust by the universal forces of gravity and friction. It takes the skilled hands and intelligence of a master watchmaker, who is intelligent and very much alive, to assemble and build a watch. How ridiculously simple is the finest watch in comparison to the most simple form of life.

Intensified effort revealed that even the supposedly simple amoeba was a complex, self-operating chemical factory. The notion that he was a simple blob, the discovery of whose chemical composition would enable us

6. James Reston, The New York *Times,* November 13, 1966, p. 6E.

instantly to set the life process in operation, turned out
to be, at best, a monstrous caricature of the truth.[7]

Innate forces are constantly at work in every living cell,
using the simple universal forces and simple universal elements to *construct* more complicated matter, maintain it,
improve it, and reproduce it. The universal forces are constantly disassembling or tearing down matter, while the living
innate forces are constantly building up matter.

When we as chiropractors understand all the above words
and what they mean, we are humbled and staggered by the
awesome complexity of human life. Sixty trillion highly
specialized living cells are working in harmony for the benefit
of one person as one whole living unit. The most complex of
all living cells is the nerve cell. All the actions, reactions and
adaptations necessary for life are caused by the conduction of
the innate intelligence to and from all areas of the body by 10
billion nerve cells.

> ... early in the Embryo the integrating instrument is the
> nervous system which constitutes the *primary* mechanism
> of physiological control and co-ordination [italics mine].[8]

Since an abnormally functioning spinal column interferes
with the transmission of the life-giving intelligence, it is a
fearful responsibility of chiropractors to remove those inter-
ferences. The responsibility is immense, because if one
changes the spine from the normal or makes it less normal
than one finds it, one is guilty of taking away some degree of
life in that person. However, if one is mindful of one's
responsibility, properly educated in one's philosophy, science,

7. Eiseley, *The Immense Journey,* p. 92.
8. Leslie Brainer Arey, Ph.D., Sc.D., Ll.D., *Developmental Anatomy* (Philadelphia: W. B. Saunders Co., 1954), pp. 24, 25.

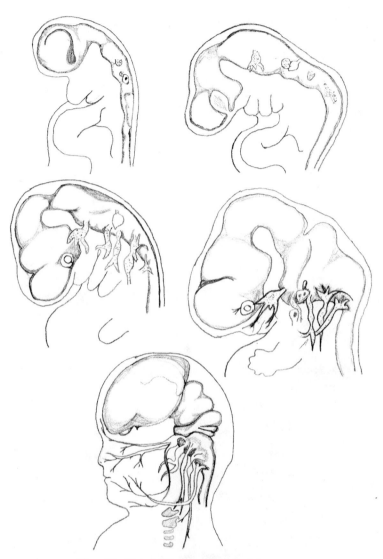

Fig. 19. Fetal life is controlled by nerves.

and art, and able to skillfully remove the nerve interference, one will be an outstanding professional, giving life to the dying.

What in God's world could be better than that?

Instead of being bent on the alteration and destruction of the environment, man must learn to come into harmony with it.[9]

9. Richard G. Van Gelder, *Animal Kingdom* (New York: The Danbury Press, Grolier Enterprises, 1972).

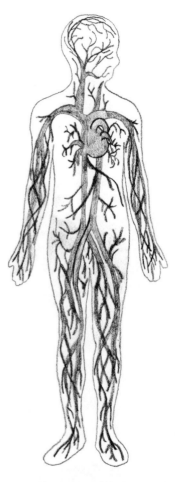
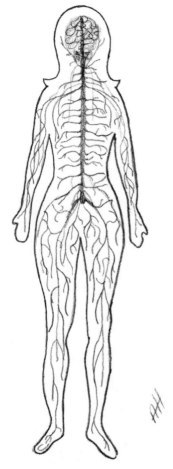

Life is built up by food   Life is organized by mental
from the blood.   impulses over nerves.

Fig. 20. Life is built up by food from the blood and organized by
mental impulses over the nerves.

103

BIBLIOGRAPHY

Arey, Leslie Brainer, Ph.D., Sc.D., Ll.D., *Developmental Anatomy* Philadelphia; W. B. Saunders Co., 1954.

Bach, Marcus, Ph.D., *The Chiropractic Story*, Los Angeles: DeVorss & Co., 1968.

Bryan, Arthur H., and Charles G., Ph.Ds., *Bacteriology, Principles and Practice,* New York: Barnes & Noble Books, 1938.

Cailliet, Rene, M.D., *Low Back Pain Syndrome,* Philadelphia; F. A. Davis Co., 1962.

Cannon, Walter B., M.D., Sc.D., *The Wisdom of the Body,* New York: W. W. Norton & Co., Inc., 1967.

Cherrington, Sir Charles, *Integrative Action of the Nervous System,* New Haven, Conn.: Yale University Press, 1947.

Chrane, V. B., D.C., Ph.C., *Health Within Your Reach,* Montgomery, Ala.: The Chiropractic Layman's League, Inc., 1970.

Discovery, Peabody Museum of Natural History, New Haven, Conn.: Yale University Press, May, 1962.

Dorland's Medical Dictionary, Philadelphia: W. B. Saunders Co., 1957.

Durant, Will, Ph.D., *The Story of Philosophy,* New York: Washington Square Press, 1961.

Dye, A. A., D.C. Ph.C., *The Evolution of Chiropractic,* Philadelphia: A. A. Dye, 1939.

Eiseley, Loren, *The Immense Journey,* New York: Random House, Inc., 1957.

Gray, Henry, *Gray's Anatomy*, Philadelphia: Lea & Febiger, 1954.

Gray, Sir James, *Science Today,* Great Britain, Granada TV Network, 1960.

Hawkes, Jacquetta, Ph.D., *Man on Earth*, New York: Random House, Inc., 1954.

Kelly, Florence C., M.S., Ph.D., and Hite, K. Eileen, Ph.D., M.D., *Microbiology*, New York: Appleton-Century-Crofts, 1955.

Jackson, Ruth, B.A., M.D., F.A.C.S., *The Cervical Syndrome*, Springfield, Ill.: Charles C Thomas, 1965.

Janse, Joseph, D.C., Houser, R. H., D.C., and Wells, B. F., D.O., D.C., *Chiropractic Principles and Technic*, Chicago: National College of Chiropractic, 1947.

Lovett, Robert W., M.D., *Lateral Curvature of the Spine*, Philadelphia: P. Blakiston Son and Co., 1916.

Moore, Ruth, B.A., M.A., *Evolution*, New York: Life Nature Library, Time-Life Books, 1964.

Ovenden, Michael W., Ph.D., *Life in the Universe*, Garden City, N.Y.: Anchor Books, Doubleday & Company, Inc., 1962.

Palmer, B. J., D.C., Ph.C., *History Repeats*, Davenport, Iowa: The Palmer School of Chiropractic, 1951; *It Is As Simple As That*, Davenport, Iowa: the Palmer School of Chiropractic, 1946; *The B. J. Palmer Chiropractic Clinic* Volume XX, Davenport, Iowa: The Palmer School of Chiropractic, 1938; *The Science of Chiropractic Its Principles and Philosophies* Volume I, Davenport, Iowa: The Palmer School of Chiropractic, 1920.

Palmer, D. D., D.C., Ph.C., *The Chiropractor*, Los Angeles: Press of Beacon Light Printing Co., 1914.

Pharaoh, Donald O., D.C., Ph.C., *Chiropractic Orthopedy*, Davenport, Iowa: The Palmer School of Chiropractic, 1956.

Reston, James, The New York *Times*, November 12, 1966.

Rodale, J. I., *The Synonym Finder*, Emmaus, Pa.: Rodale Books, 1961.

Rodale, Robert, Chicago Tribune Syndicate *Organic Living*, Eugene, Oregon: Emerald Empire Magazine, p. 18, Eugene *Register Guard*, April 15, 1973.

Science Year, Chicago: Field Enterprises Educational Corp., 1965.

Stephenson, Ralph W., D.C., Ph.C., *Chiropractic Textbook*, Davenport, Iowa: The Palmer School of Chiropractic, 1927.

Stonebrink, R. D., B.S., D.C., F.I.C.C., *Basic Features of Subluxation and the Principles and Practice of Chiropractic*, Portland, Oregon: Western States College of Chiropractic, 1972.

Szent-Gyorgyi, Albert, M.D., Ph.D., *The Crazy Ape*, New York: Grosset & Dunlap, 1970.

Taber, Clarence Wilbur, *Taber's Cyclopedic Medical Dictionary*, Philadelphia: F.A. Davis Co., 1952.

Tanner, James M., and Taylor, Gordon Rattray, *Growth*, New York: Life Science Library, Time-Life Books, 1965.

The Illustrated Encyclopedia of Animal Kingdom, Volume I, New York: The Danbury Press, Grolier Enterprises, 1972.

Villee, Claude A., Ph.D., *Biology*, Philadelphia: W. B. Saunders Co., 1954.

Webster's New Collegiate Dictionary, Springfield, Mass.; G. & C. Merriam Co., 1953.

Weidenreich, Franz, Ph.D., *Apes, Giants, and Man*, Chicago: The University of Chicago Press, 1956.

Wilson, John Rowan, M.D., and Editors of Life, *The Mind*, New York: Life Science Library, Time-Life Books, 1961.

World Book Encyclopedia, Chicago: Field Enterprises Educational Corp. 1964.